PHOTOTHERAPY
TREATMENT PROTOCOLS

Series in Dermatological Treatment

Series editors

Steven R Feldman

and

Peter van de Kerkhof

Published in association with the *Journal of Dermatological Treatment*

PHOTOTHERAPY
TREATMENT PROTOCOLS

THIRD EDITION

The methods of

Steven R. Feldman M.D., Ph.D.
Wake Forest University School of Medicine
Winston-Salem, NC, USA

and

Michael D. Zanolli M.D.
Nashville, TN, USA
Past President of The Photomedicine Society

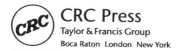

CRC Press
Taylor & Francis Group
Boca Raton London New York

CRC Press is an imprint of the
Taylor & Francis Group, an **informa** business

CRC Press
Taylor & Francis Group
6000 Broken Sound Parkway NW, Suite 300
Boca Raton, FL 33487-2742

© 2016 by Taylor & Francis Group, LLC
CRC Press is an imprint of Taylor & Francis Group, an Informa business

No claim to original U.S. Government works

Printed on acid-free paper
Version Date: 20160510

International Standard Book Number-13: 978-1-4987-5462-0 (Paperback)

Visit the Taylor & Francis Web site at
http://www.taylorandfrancis.com

and the CRC Press Web site at
http://www.crcpress.com

TABLE OF CONTENTS

ACKNOWLEDGMENTS

The authors thank terrific dedicated phototherapists Bobbie Oliver, Sharon Sharp, Beverly Webb, and Barbara Brown, RN, for their advice and skillful, compassionate care of patients. The efforts of the National Psoriasis Foundation on behalf of all our patients with psoriasis cannot go unnoticed. Finally, the authors thank Taylor & Francis Group for their tireless support in the development of this manual.

INTRODUCTION TO THE THIRD EDITION

The treatment of psoriasis has evolved dramatically since the last edition. The introduction of tumor necrosis factor inhibitors revolutionized the treatment of psoriasis. Then came an interleukin-12/interleukin-23 inhibitor that only requires one injection every 3 months, about equal in efficacy to the strongest of the tumor necrosis factor inhibitors. And now, in interleukin-17 inhibitors, we have even more potent treatments. Moreover, the safety of these new systemic treatments knocks the socks off the former gold-standard systemic treatments of the past, methotrexate and cyclosporine.

But biologics are expensive and should only be used in patients who need them. For patients with psoriasis or other diseases that can be effectively treated with phototherapy, biologics may not be required. In an era of constantly increasing focus on reducing the cost of disease management, phototherapy—which has fallen to the side in the wake of biologic excitement—may be poised for resurgence. The array of phototherapy options—from whole body and targeted phototherapy in the office to home phototherapy—remain a valuable, effective, safe, and cost-effective way to manage a host of skin conditions.

We hope this manual helps give you the tools you need to make phototherapy more accessible to your patients.

Steven R. Feldman

INTRODUCTION TO THE SECOND EDITION

The basic premise concerning the therapeutic option of phototherapy remains the same for the second edition as with our first edition. The first sentence of the introduction to the first edition reads: "The availability of phototherapy in a dermatology practice enables the practitioner to provide a broader range of therapeutic options." I encourage the persons utilizing the protocols contained in this book to read through the Introduction to the First Edition to enable them to have a better understanding of the application of therapeutic ultraviolet light therapy for inflammatory diseases. The continued modifications of protocols, although minimal in most circumstances, demonstrate the ongoing refinement of ultraviolet light delivery to maintain therapeutic efficacy while minimizing possible side effects.

New delivery systems for ultraviolet light, whether in the form of laser or localized ultraviolet B light, have been an advancement in the application of phototherapy for the same diseases that are treated with whole body phototherapy. The incorporation of protocols for localized delivery enables even more utility for treatment with ultraviolet light to the affected areas while sparing the clinically normal skin. The localized delivery technology brings with it a shift in the approach to treatment. Instead of limiting the dose energy delivered to the whole body in order to minimize the possible side effects of ultraviolet light to uninvolved skin, the areas to be treated are given multiples of the minimal erythema dose to produce the most rapid and effective clearing of the diseased skin. In addition, while treating specialized diseases such as vitiligo with localized ultraviolet light, the dose can be adjusted to use lower amounts of light to depigmented areas without enhancing the contrast with surrounding normal skin. The addition of protocols using localized delivery of ultraviolet light is an important aspect of this new second edition.

The effects of ultraviolet light on the skin continue to be a source of new insight into the physiology and pathophysiology as related to the broader field of photobiology and photomedicine. I remain fascinated by the continued developments in this field that help us to understand why ultraviolet light is such a beneficial therapy for inflammatory dermatosis of the skin. There are clearly differences in the effects in the skin with delivery of high-dose ultraviolet light at various wavelengths when compared to lower doses of ultraviolet light. As with the more recent advent of protein immune modifiers for the treatment of psoriasis, the "biologics," the effects of ultraviolet light in low doses serve to modify the skin's immune mechanisms and help decrease the activity of psoriasis. Further insights into the complex interactive pathways of the cutaneous immune system will not only help to refine therapeutic intervention but will also add to the understanding of the pathophysiology of the disease. Use of these protocols for treatment of responsive skin diseases is in effect application of "photobiologic" therapy. The continued use of ultraviolet light by medical specialists will remain an option for therapeutic intervention for chronic inflammatory skin diseases.

Michael D. Zanolli
Steven R. Feldman

The availability of phototherapy in a dermatology practice enables the practitioner to provide a broader range of therapeutic options. This is especially true for those dermatologists who treat a large number of inflammatory dermatoses, particularly psoriasis. The development of a phototherapy unit, even if it is just a single ultraviolet light cabinet, will serve not only the patients in a particular practice, but can also serve as a regional referral center. Smaller communities surrounding such a location would tend to refer to a local center rather than having the patients undertake time-consuming drives two or three times a week for phototherapy at a less convenient site in a large urban setting.

There are many textbooks concerning photomedicine, photobiology, and therapeutic applications for ultraviolet light (see Suggested Reading). These are invaluable for understanding the scientific underpinning of phototherapy and the development of the protocols contained in this manual. The expertise of the physician concerning the proper delivery of ultraviolet light treatments for a particular patient or a particular disease is essential to obtaining the best outcomes. The physician should also serve as the resource for information concerning medical aspects of phototherapy. This manual provides a practical basis for phototherapy protocols and consent forms that can be modified or adjusted by the physician to meet the specific needs of specific patients.

In addition to the important role played by the physician in determining treatment regimens, special training on the part of the phototherapy nurses and technicians has become more important for the continuity of care and for determining the standard of care for any particular region. Essential to any phototherapy location are the expert nursing efforts necessary to carry through the implementation of the protocols and to be vigilant for signs, especially early subtle signs, of phototoxic reactions and other possible side effects during the course of therapy. Physicians should strongly consider the benefits of using another practical resource for psoriasis patient education: the National Psoriasis Foundation.

The genesis and development of this phototherapy manual occurred because of the need to have available on site a standard of the protocols for delivery of medical treatments for compliance with local and federal regulations. This is particularly true for a hospital-based phototherapy treatment center. This compilation of treatment protocols is not meant to be absolute, comprehensive, or construed as the only method for delivery of care. The protocols continue to be in a state of development and modification to better improve the response to therapy and, it is hoped, to decrease the frequency of side effects. Another factor that enters into the modifications of phototherapy protocols is the advent of newer technology, such as narrowband UVB or the use of psoralen medications other than 8-methoxypsoralen in the future. The use of phototherapy and enhancement of therapeutic response must always take into consideration the risk of side effects from the particular modality of treatment, both short and long term.

The original protocol manual was devised at the Bowman-Gray School of Medicine, Wake Forest University Medical Center, for its Psoriasis Day Care Center in 1986. Many changes in the overall treatment of psoriasis have occurred since that time, such as outpatient Goeckerman treatment being used much less frequently than 10 years ago. The new treatments include use of systemic retinoids, immunosuppressive treatments, and topical vitamin D_3 analogues and retinoids, often in combination with phototherapy. There are still centers at which the Goeckerman or modified Ingram treatments for psoriasis are the mainstay of their facilities. However, more outpatient treatments and increased use of combination therapy with ultraviolet light and topical therapy or ultraviolet light and systemic therapy bring the outpatient treatment of psoriasis back to dermatologists' offices. This eliminates the need for large outlays of capital for the development of treatment centers that would occupy 1000–1500 ft^2 in order to provide the facilities necessary for day-care treatments, bath facilities, lounge areas, and multiple treatment rooms.

This text is meant to be an office-based manual that can be used as the office procedure manual. It can be referred to on a daily basis by the phototherapy technicians, as well as used as a resource if any questions arise about the standards of care within an office. We encourage you to make and modify copies of the consent forms and other documents and use them for patients in your practice.

This manual is not meant to be a rigid text. The protocols have undergone and continue to undergo their own genesis. Modifications or additions to the text for delivery of ultraviolet light for a particular disease or variations between skin types that best suit the practitioner can be done to the main body of the text with minimal effort. The manual also can be used as a basis for treatment of photoresponsive diseases that are not individually listed or do not have sections devoted to them. Other entities reported in dermatological literature as responsive to ultraviolet light therapy would include eosinophilic folliculitis, granuloma annulare, graft vs. host disease, certain forms of lichen planus, and, of course, variations on the parapsoriasis group of disorders, such as large plaque parapsoriasis and/or common pityriasis rosea. The basis for treatment of these disorders and necessary protocols for the phototherapy technicians or nurses to follow can be derived by the local site and kept on file for reference.

One of the basic principles to be understood when selecting ultraviolet therapy, whether in the form of UVB or photochemotherapy with PUVA, is each disease entity may not and should not be treated exactly alike. The phototherapy for psoriasis differs from the approach to therapy for a mild case of pityriasis rosea. In general, phototherapy can be therapeutic even when used in a nonerythemogenic modality, and this is particularly true when dealing with forms of photochemotherapy. Therefore, the manual has extreme flexibility, and the most common of the photoresponsive dermatoses are listed with fairly specific protocols that have been used for the past 14 years with methods that have been modified through experience and found to be successful. Other dermatoses may also be treated with a different dosage and frequency of therapy for a specific disorder. For example, the treatment modality for atopic dermatitis with UVA/UVB combination therapy may also be used to treat eosinophilic folliculitis. The protocol for treatment of generalized granuloma annulare may also be adopted from the treatment protocol used for cutaneous T-cell lymphoma. The understanding and the insights into the photobiology associated with the changes of improvement in the inflammatory dermatoses are also going to continue to be more delineated as time goes on. This manual can serve as the source of defined protocols for the delivery of therapeutic ultraviolet light and can be modified to treat those other dermatoses that may not be corticosteroid responsive, without the need for systemic immunosuppressive therapy in many cases.

The development and modifications of this manual, initially at Wake Forest University Medical Center, then at the Vanderbilt Phototherapy Treatment Center, have only been possible and brought to light because of the continuing efforts of the dedicated physicians and personnel at both institutions. The requests of practicing dermatologists for such a manual have been the moving force behind getting this project to the dermatology community. More important are the benefits to the patients who can now receive phototherapy closer to home and through their own dermatologists' offices. The overall use of phototherapy as an office procedure can be very rewarding for practitioners because of the broad range of dermatoses that have been reported as being responsive to therapeutic intervention with ultraviolet light treatment. In my opinion, the gratification of being able to deliver a therapeutic option, which is so beneficial to patients with photoresponsive dermatoses, will make providing such treatment a satisfying part of any busy dermatology practice.

Michael D. Zanolli

WARNING

Narrowband UVB protocols use more energy (joules) than broadband protocols. *Do not* use the narrowband protocols with broadband equipment as serious harm could result.

National Psoriasis Foundation

Dermatologists offering phototherapy should keep in mind the National Psoriasis Foundation (NPF), a terrific resource for our psoriasis patients. The NPF has great patient education resources, with a wide variety of brochures available free (digitally) to doctors to help educate patients about phototherapy and their other treatment options. It supports the specialty of dermatology by working with insurers and regulators to assure patients have access to dermatologists and to psoriasis treatments. The Foundation can also help with a critical issue for dermatologists setting up a phototherapy unit: the education of the phototherapist through NPF-sponsored courses. The NPF has been an invaluable resource to the editors of this book.

The Foundation's resources are freely accessible at www.psoriasis.org. We encourage all health care professionals caring for patients with psoriasis to joint the Foundation as professional members.

PHOTOTHERAPY TREATMENT CENTER INITIAL INTRODUCTION

1. Patient referral and entry

   a. All patients must be evaluated by a dermatologist.

   b. The diagnosis must be discussed with the patient by a physician prior to referral to the phototherapy treatment center (PTC) for consultation regarding treatment options or orientation.

   c. All patients referred for treatment of any kind must have a diagnosis and designation of a skin type. See Appendices.

   d. All patients referred with the diagnosis of psoriasis will have an appointment for a consultation with the director of the PTC prior to selection of a treatment protocol.

   e. All patients with a diagnosis of photodermatosis referred for diagnostic phototesting will have an appointment for a consultation with the director of the PTC prior to initiation of phototesting procedures, except for the determination of a minimal erythema dose (MED) per the UVB or narrowband UVB (NBUVB) protocol using MED.

2. Orientation to the PTC

   a. General information
      i. All patients are to be given a tour of the PTC to include the following:
         A. Nurses' station
         B. Checking-in procedure at the nurses' station lounge/kitchen area
         C. Phototherapy rooms, scalp/treatment rooms, bathroom
         D. Lockers, bath/shower

   b. Phototherapy
      i. All patients entered into the PTC for any type of phototherapy will need the basic introduction to phototherapy in addition to specific information included with each protocol (see individual protocols).
      ii. The phototherapy equipment will be shown to the patient with special attention to the safety features of each light box or device.
      iii. All phototherapy patients will be told they must wear protective eye shields provided by the PTC.
      iv. Males must wear protection over their genitalia unless specified by the physician responsible for their care.
      v. A list of all current medications the patient is using will be placed on the chart.

   c. Hydrotherapy
      i. Specific instructions for hydrosound therapy are included in the protocol section.
      ii. Patients will be shown the hydrosound baths and the alarm system in each tub room.

      iii. All patients referred for hydrosound therapy must be able to independently stand upright when the patient lift is used to lower the patient into the bath.

3.   Consent forms

    a.   All patients who are to receive any form of phototherapy must sign a consent form that is to remain in the chart. See Section II Consent Forms (page 147).

4.   Monitoring of treatments

    a.   To ensure adequate monitoring of the patient response and timely adjustment of the dose/frequency of phototherapy, every patient undergoing phototherapy treatment should be seen by the attending physician every six to eight treatments.

    b.   Exceptions to the aforementioned rule would include patients on maintenance phototherapy for vitiligo or intractable pruritus, who should be seen every 10 treatments.

    c.   The attending physician is responsible for verifying the phototherapy record for each of their patients. This is best done on a daily basis. The phototherapy record will be kept in the PTC at all times.

Psoriasis

ULTRAVIOLET B PHOTOTHERAPY BY MINIMAL ERYTHEMA DOSE

PATIENT INSTRUCTIONS

1. All patients designated for the ultraviolet B (UVB) by minimal erythema dose (MED) protocol will have the routine introduction to the Phototherapy Treatment Center (PTC) facility.

2. All patients designated for the UVB by MED protocol will have the basic introduction to phototherapy equipment and safety procedures.

3. Reinforcement of the need for eye protection and covering of the genital area in males is required.

4. All patients with the diagnosis of psoriasis will be told to apply mineral oil to the involved areas of the skin prior to the delivery of UVB.

5. Patients are to stand in the center of the light cabinet with their arms at rest. A step stool may be used for the patients to stand on when recommended by the physician.

6. A handheld timer will be set by the phototherapy technician for each treatment session. The time will correspond to the estimated time of the treatment session duration, and the timer will either be given to the patient to have with them during the treatment session or be kept by the technician during the treatment. The time will correspond with the amount of time calculated for their dose of UVB for that treatment.

7. Instruct patients to come out of the light box when the lights have gone out or within 10 seconds of the alarm of the safety (handheld) timer. Inform patients that the light-box doors are not locked and demonstrate their operation.

8. The list of current medications will be placed in the patient's chart and reviewed by the phototherapist. Questions concerning the current medications will be addressed by the attending physician.

9. All patients will be told of the possible complications of UVB phototherapy specifically including

    a. Sunburn reaction
    b. Corneal burn if the eyes are unprotected
    c. Photoallergic dermatitis (including drug reaction)
    d. Freckling of the skin
    e. Aging of the skin
    f. Possible increase in risk of skin cancers

10. Patients will be told that additional unprotected sun exposure should be avoided on the days they receive UVB. Sunblock (SPF 15) should be used on any sun-exposed areas for the remainder of that day.

11. All patients will be given the brochure on UVB phototherapy from the National Psoriasis Foundation.

PROTOCOL

1. Obtain a signed consent form after the patient has been given the tour of the PTC and basic phototherapy education concerning UVB phototherapy. The patient should be given time for questions.

2. Obtain an MED using the standard procedure. See the section "Procedure for Determination of the MED for UVB."

3. Have the patient undress completely and apply mineral oil to areas of psoriasis prior to the treatment. Male patients should wear an athletic supporter unless otherwise directed or permitted by the attending physician.

4. Eye protection in the form of UV goggles must be worn by all patients when inside the phototherapy unit.

5. The irradiance (mW/cm^2) of the UVB light inside the unit should be recorded on a once-a-month basis using the standard method of the manufacturer of the phototherapy unit. Record this irradiance on the phototherapy record sheet or keep an irradiance logbook for the equipment used in patient care.

6. The initial UVB dose (mJ/cm^2) will be based on the patient's MED determination at 24 hours from the delivery of the test doses. The MED will be included in the phototherapy treatment record.

$$\text{Initial UVB} = 50\% \text{ of the MED}$$

   (If the patient's MED is higher than the highest dose of UVB delivered in the MED determination testing, then a dose of 50% of the highest test site will be used as the initial dose.)

7. The manual method for calculation of the time (seconds) to set the UVB control panel to deliver the dose from #6 is the following equation: (The measurement of the irradiance can be obtained from the logbook kept on a weekly basis.)

$$\text{Time (seconds)} = \text{Dose (mJ/cm}^2\text{)} \div \text{Irradiance (mW/cm}^2\text{)}$$

8. The duration of a treatment or total dose of UVB to be delivered can often be calculated by the ultraviolet (UV) light unit by following the manufacturer's instructions in the operations manual and inputting the correct information on the control panel prior to the delivery of the treatment.

9. Set the time (or dose) on the control panel of the UV light unit and on the additional safety timer kept in the light unit or by the technician. In some phototherapy units, the session duration is dependent on the dose measured by an internal photometer, and the time must be estimated by the technician.

10. Verify that the UV light unit is set on UVB.

11. Turn on the fan and have the patient stand in the center of the UV light unit with their arms at rest. Double-check that they are wearing UV goggles as eye protection.

12. Instruct the patient to come out of the UV light box when the lights go out or if they become uncomfortable during the treatment either from burning or stinging of the skin. Inform the patient that the light-box doors are not locked.

13. Start the treatment.

SUBSEQUENT TREATMENTS

14. The frequency of UVB using MED light treatments for the diagnosis of psoriasis is 3–5 times a week unless otherwise ordered by a physician. If less than 3 times a week has been ordered by a physician, then special instructions for the advancement of the dose of UVB light must accompany the request.

15. On subsequent visits, the patient will be asked about redness, light pink color, and tenderness of the skin the previous night, and this information will be put into the phototherapy record.

16. If the skin is a light pink color, the phototherapist should keep the dose the same as the previously delivered treatment dose.

17. If the skin is red, the phototherapy technician will ask that the patient be seen by the attending physician who will make the decision for adjustment in the UVB treatment.

18. Increase the dose (mJ/cm^2) of the UVB light by the amount as follows, and add it to the previous dose delivered to the patient if the treatment has been within 3 days:

Treatments 1–10	Increase by 25% of the MED.
Treatments 11–20	Increase by 10% of the MED.
Treatments 21–X	Increase as ordered by physician.

19. For subsequent treatments, these corresponding steps can be done if the following time between treatments have been observed:

4–7 days	Keep the dose the same.
1–2 weeks	Decrease the dose by 25%.
2–4 weeks	Decrease the dose by 50%.
More than 4 weeks	Start over.

20. Follow steps 7–13 previously.

MAINTENANCE THERAPY FOR UVB

Once there has been acceptable improvement in the severity of the psoriasis, patients may be kept on intermittent treatments as a maintenance therapy. There is great variability in selection of the optimal frequency and dose of UVB needed to keep an acceptable control of psoriasis. The following general guidelines may be used:

If psoriasis has cleared (>75%), the following guidelines can be considered:

Once a week treatments for 4 weeks	Keep the dose the same.
Once every 2 weeks long term	Decrease the dose by 25% and hold.

The activity of the underlying psoriatic condition may require long-term maintenance therapy, especially during the winter months or in locations of northern latitudes. If there has been an acceptable response (75%–100% clearance), then maintenance therapy at once every 2 weeks can be continued to keep the activity of the psoriasis under control in many patients. Long-term therapy, whether in the form of combination therapy or systemic therapy, would need to be discussed between the patient and physician. For those patients responding to and requiring long-term maintenance UVB, a home UVB or NBUVB unit may warrant consideration.

PROCEDURE FOR DETERMINATION OF THE MED FOR UVB

1. Prior to the initiation of phototherapy treatments, the patient will be asked to attend the treatment center for 2 consecutive days.

2. The area to be tested is to be a sun-protected region on the hip or buttocks.

3. Other areas of the skin must be covered with layers of cloth over clothing or UV protective material.

4. The ports to be irradiated should be uniform in size and at least 2 cm^2.

5. Specific garments for MED determinations with eight or more ports should be used for the phototesting.

6. The location of each port should be identified by a lateral ink mark or some other type of identification for localization of the areas tested.

7. The dose for each port for routine UVB phototesting is dependent on the skin type of the person to be tested. The two dosage schedules are as follows:

Skin Types I–III (mJ/cm^2)	Skin Types IV–VI (mJ/cm^2)
A. 20	A. 60
B. 30	B. 70
C. 40	C. 80
D. 50	D. 90
E. 60	E. 100
F. 80	F. 120

8.   The patient is to wear eye protection during the delivery of the UV doses for the MED testing.

9.   The dosage delivery can best be done by beginning with all of the ports open for UV testing and closing the individual ports after a specific dose of UV light has been delivered.

10. At the completion of the phototesting, the special garments used in the testing should be removed, and the areas rechecked to make sure adequate marking of the skin has been done to identify the actual ports tested.

11. The patient will be instructed to avoid any natural or artificial UV light to this region of the skin during the next 24 hours.

12. The patient is to return to the phototherapy center in 24 hours.

13. The area of the phototesting should be identified by the markings at the different dosage sites.

14. Identifiable erythema within the margins of the phototesting port is considered a positive reading.

15. If bright red erythema develops or blistering occurs at the site of any of the phototesting sites, then topical corticosteroids can be used to treat the area.

ULTRAVIOLET B PHOTOTHERAPY BY SKIN TYPE

PATIENT INSTRUCTIONS

1. All patients designated for the UVB protocol will have the routine introduction to the PTC facility.

2. All patients designated for the UVB protocol will have the basic introduction to phototherapy equipment and safety procedures.

3. Reinforcement of the need for eye protection and covering of the genital area in males is required.

4. All patients with the diagnosis of psoriasis will be told to apply mineral oil to the involved areas of the skin prior to the delivery of UVB.

5. Patients are to stand in the center of the light cabinet with their arms at rest. A step stool may be used for the patients to stand on when recommended by the physician.

6. A handheld timer will be set by the phototherapy technician for each treatment session. The time will correspond to the estimated time of the treatment session duration, and the timer will either be given to the patients to have with them during the treatment session or be kept by the technician during the treatment. The time will correspond with the amount of time calculated for their dose of UVB for that treatment.

7. Instruct patients to come out of the light box when the lights have gone out or within 10 seconds of the alarm of the safety (handheld) timer. Inform patients that the light-box doors are not locked and demonstrate their operation.

8. The list of current medications will be placed in the patient's chart and reviewed by the phototherapist. Questions concerning the current medications will be addressed by the attending physician.

9. All patients will be told of the possible complications of UVB phototherapy specifically including

    a. Sunburn reaction
    b. Corneal burn if the eyes are unprotected
    c. Photoallergic dermatitis (including drug reaction)
    d. Freckling of the skin
    e. Aging of the skin
    f. Possible increase in risk of skin cancers

10. Patients will be told that additional unprotected sun exposure should be avoided on the days they receive UVB. Sunblock (SPF 15) should be used on any sun-exposed areas for the remainder of that day.

11. All patients will be given the brochure on UVB phototherapy from the National Psoriasis Foundation.

PROTOCOL

1. Obtain a signed consent form after the patient has been given the tour of the PTC and basic phototherapy education concerning UVB phototherapy. The patient should be given time for questions.

2. Have the patient undress completely. Male patients should wear an athletic supporter unless otherwise directed or permitted by the attending physician. Patients will apply mineral oil on the plaques of psoriasis prior to the delivery of UV light.

3. Eye protection in the form of UV goggles must be worn by all patients when inside the phototherapy unit.

4. The irradiance (mW/cm^2) of the UVB light inside the unit should be recorded on a once-a-month basis using the standard method of the manufacturer of the phototherapy unit. Record this irradiance on the phototherapy record sheet or keep an irradiance logbook for the equipment used in patient care.

5. Determine the initial UVB dose (mJ/cm^2) according to the patient's skin type as classified by the physician. See Appendix for definitions of skin types.

Skin Type	Initial UVB Dose (mJ/cm^2)
Type I	20
Type II	25
Type III	30
Type IV	40
Type V	50
Type VI	60

6. The manual method for calculation of the time (seconds) to set the UVB control panel to deliver the dose from #5 is the following equation: (The measurement of the irradiance can be obtained from the logbook kept on a weekly basis.)

$$\text{Time (seconds)} = \text{Dose (mJ/cm}^2) \div \text{Irradiance (mW/cm}^2)$$

7. The duration of a treatment or total dose of UVB to be delivered can often be calculated electronically by the UV light unit by following the manufacturer's instructions in the operations manual and inputting the correct information on the control panel prior to the delivery of the treatment.

8. Set the time (or dose) on the control panel of the UV light unit and on the additional safety timer kept in the light unit or by the technician. In some phototherapy units, the session duration is dependent on the dose measured by an internal photometer, and the time must be estimated by the technician.

9. Verify that the UV light unit is set on UVB.

8

10. Turn on the fan and have the patient stand in the center of the ultraviolet light unit with their arms at rest. Double-check that they are wearing UV goggles as eye protection.

11. Instruct the patient to come out of the UV light box when the lights go out or if they become uncomfortable during the treatment either from burning or stinging of the skin. Inform the patient that the light-box doors are not locked.

12. Start the treatment.

SUBSEQUENT TREATMENTS

13. The frequency of UVB light treatments for the diagnosis of psoriasis is 3–5 times a week unless otherwise ordered by a physician. If less than 3 times a week has been ordered by a physician, then special instructions for the advancement of the dose of UVB light must accompany the request.

14. On subsequent visits, the patient will be asked about redness, light pink color, and tenderness of the skin the previous night, and this information will be put into the phototherapy record.

15. If the skin is red, the phototherapist will ask that the patient be seen by the attending physician who will make the decision for adjustment in the UVB treatment. If the skin is a light pink color, the phototherapist should keep the dose the same as the previously delivered dose.

16. Increase the dose (mJ/cm^2) of the UVB light by the amount as follows and add it to the previous dose delivered to the patient if the treatment has been within 3 days:

Skin Type	Amount of UVB Increase (mJ/cm^2)
Type I	5
Type II	10
Type III	15
Type IV	20
Type V	25
Type VI	30

17. For subsequent treatments, if the following time between treatments have been observed, these corresponding steps can be done:

4–7 days	Keep the dose the same.
1–2 weeks	Decrease the dose by 50%.
2–3 weeks	Decrease the dose by 75%.
3 or more weeks	Start over.

18. Follow steps 6–12 previously.

MAINTENANCE THERAPY FOR UVB

Once there has been acceptable improvement in the severity of the psoriasis, patients may be kept on intermittent treatments as a maintenance therapy. There is great variability in selection of the optimal frequency and dose of UVB needed to keep an acceptable control of psoriasis. The following general guidelines may be used:

If psoriasis has cleared (>75%), consider the following guidelines:

Once a week treatments for 4 weeks	Keep the dose the same.
Once every 2 weeks long term	Decrease the dose by 25% and hold.

The activity of the underlying psoriatic condition may require long-term maintenance therapy, especially during the winter months or in locations of northern latitudes. If there has been an acceptable response (75%–100% clearance), then maintenance therapy at once every 2 weeks can be continued to keep the activity of the psoriasis under control in many patients. Long-term therapy, whether in the form of combination therapy or systemic therapy, would need to be discussed between the patient and physician. For those patients responding to and requiring long-term maintenance UVB, a home UVB or NBUVB unit may warrant consideration.

NARROWBAND ULTRAVIOLET B PHOTOTHERAPY BY MED

PATIENT INSTRUCTIONS

1. All patients designated for the narrowband ultraviolet B (NBUVB) by MED protocol will have the routine introduction to the PTC facility.

2. All patients designated for the NBUVB by MED protocol will have the basic introduction to phototherapy equipment and safety procedures.

3. Reinforcement of the need for eye protection and covering of the genital area in males is required.

4. Patients are to stand in the center of the light cabinet with their arms at rest. A step stool may be used for the patients to stand on when recommended by the physician.

5. A handheld timer will be set by the phototherapy technician for each treatment session. The time will correspond to the estimated time of the treatment session duration, and the timer will either be given to the patient to have with them during the treatment session or be kept by the technician during the treatment. The time will correspond with the amount of time calculated for their dose of NBUVB for that treatment.

6. Instruct patients to come out of the light box when the lights have gone out or within 10 seconds of the alarm of the safety (handheld) timer. Inform patients that the light-box doors are not locked and demonstrate their operation.

7. The list of current medications will be placed in the patient's chart and reviewed by the phototherapist. Questions concerning the current medications will be addressed by the attending physician.

8. All patients will be told of the possible complications of NBUVB phototherapy specifically including

    a. Sunburn reaction
    b. Corneal burn if the eyes are unprotected
    c. Photoallergic dermatitis (including drug reaction)
    d. Freckling of the skin
    e. Aging of the skin
    f. Possible increase in risk of skin cancers

9. Patients will be told that additional unprotected sun exposure should be avoided on the days they receive NBUVB. Sunblock (SPF 15) should be used on any sun-exposed areas for the remainder of that day.

10. All patients will be given the brochure on UVB phototherapy from the National Psoriasis Foundation.

PROTOCOL

1. Obtain a signed consent form after the patient has been given the tour of the PTC and basic phototherapy education concerning NBUVB phototherapy. The patient should be given time for questions.

2. Obtain an MED using the standard procedure. See the section "Procedure for Determination of the MED for NBUVB."

3. Have the patient undress completely and apply mineral oil to areas of psoriasis prior to the treatment. Male patients should wear an athletic supporter unless otherwise directed or permitted by the attending physician.

4. Eye protection in the form of UV goggles must be worn by all patients when inside the phototherapy unit.

5. The irradiance (mW/cm^2) of the NBUVB light inside the unit should be recorded on a once-a-month basis using the standard method of the manufacturer of the phototherapy unit. Record this irradiance on the phototherapy record sheet or keep an irradiance logbook for the equipment used in patient care.

6. The initial NBUVB dose (mJ/cm^2) will be based on the patient's MED determination at 24 hours from the delivery of the test doses. The MED will be included in the phototherapy treatment record.

Initial NBUVB = 50% of the MED

(If the patient's MED is higher than the highest dose of NBUVB delivered in the MED determination testing, then a dose of 50% of the highest test site will be used as the initial dose.)

7. The manual method for calculation of the time (seconds) to set the NBUVB control panel to deliver the dose from #6 is the following equation: (The measurement of the irradiance can be obtained from the logbook kept on a weekly basis.)

$$\text{Time (seconds)} = \text{Dose (mJ/cm}^2) \div \text{Irradiance (mW/cm}^2)$$

8. The duration of a treatment or total dose of NBUVB to be delivered can often be calculated by the UV light unit by following the manufacturer's instructions in the operations manual and inputting the correct information on the control panel prior to the delivery of the treatment.

9. Set the time (or dose) on the control panel of the UV light unit and on the additional safety timer kept in the light unit or by the technician. In some phototherapy units, the session duration is dependent on the dose measured by an internal photometer, and the time must be estimated by the technician.

10. Verify that the UV light unit is set on NBUVB.

11. Turn on the fan and have the patient stand in the center of the UV light unit with their arms at rest. Double-check that they are wearing UV goggles as eye protection.

12. Instruct the patient to come out of the UV light box when the lights go out or if they become uncomfortable during the treatment either from burning or stinging of the skin. Inform the patient that the light-box doors are not locked.

13. Start the treatment.

SUBSEQUENT TREATMENTS

14. The frequency of NBUVB using MED light treatments for the diagnosis of psoriasis is 3–4 times a week unless otherwise ordered by a physician. If less than 3 times a week has been ordered by a physician, then special instructions for the advancement of the dose of NBUVB light must accompany the request.

15. On subsequent visits, the patient will be asked about redness, light pink color, and tenderness of the skin the previous night, and this information will be put into the phototherapy record.

16. If the skin is red, the phototherapy technician will ask that the patient be seen by the attending physician who will make the decision for adjustment in the NBUVB treatment. If the skin is a light pink color, the phototherapist should keep the dose the same as the previously delivered treatment dose.

17. Increase the dose (mJ/cm^2) of the NBUVB light by the amount as follows, and add it to the previous dose delivered to the patient if the treatment has been within 3 days:

Treatments 1–20	Increase by 10% of the MED.
Treatments 21–X	Increase as ordered by physician.

18. Do not exceed 4 times the MED unless otherwise ordered by the physician.

19. For subsequent treatments, here are the corresponding steps if the following time between treatments have been observed:

4–7 days	Keep the dose the same.
1–2 weeks	Decrease the dose by 25%.
2–4 weeks	Decrease the dose by 50%.
More than 4 weeks	Start over.

20. Follow steps 7–13 previously.

MAINTENANCE THERAPY FOR NBUVB

Once there has been acceptable improvement in the severity of the psoriasis, patients may be kept on intermittent treatments as a maintenance therapy. There is great variability in selection of the optimal frequency and dose of NBUVB needed to keep an acceptable control of psoriasis. The following general guidelines may be used:

If psoriasis has cleared (>75%), consider the following guidelines:

Once a week treatments for 4 weeks	Keep the dose the same.
Once every 2 weeks long term	Decrease the dose by 25% and hold.

The activity of the underlying psoriatic condition may require long-term maintenance therapy, especially during the winter months or in locations of northern latitudes. If there has been an acceptable response (75%–100% clearance), then maintenance therapy at once every 2 weeks can be continued to keep the activity of the psoriasis under control in many patients. Long-term therapy whether in the form of combination therapy or systemic therapy would need to be discussed between the patient and physician. For those patients responding to and requiring long-term maintenance UVB, a home UVB or NBUVB unit may warrant consideration.

PROCEDURE FOR DETERMINATION OF THE MED FOR NBUVB

1. Prior to the initiation of phototherapy treatments, the patient will be asked to attend the treatment center for 2 consecutive days.

2. The area to be tested is to be a sun-protected region on the hip or buttocks.

3. Other areas of the skin must be covered with layers of cloth over clothing or UV protective material.

4. The ports to be irradiated should be uniform in size and at least 2 cm^2.

5. Specific garments for MED determinations with six or more ports should be used for the phototesting.

6. The location of each port should be identified by a lateral ink mark or some other type of identification for localization of the areas tested.

7. The dose for each port for routine UVB phototesting is dependent on the skin type of the person to be tested. The two dosage schedules are as follows:

Skin Types I–III (mJ/cm^2)	Skin Types IV–VI (mJ/cm^2)
A. 400	A. 800
B. 600	B. 1000
C. 800	C. 1200
D. 1000	D. 1400
E. 1200	E. 1600
F. 1400	F. 1800

8. The patient is to wear eye protection during the delivery of the UV doses for the MED testing.

9. The dosage delivery can best be done by beginning with all of the ports open for UV testing and closing the individual ports after a specific dose of UV light has been delivered.

10. At the completion of the phototesting the special garments used in the testing should be removed and the areas rechecked to make sure adequate marking of the skin has been done to identify the actual ports tested.

11. The patient will be instructed not to receive any natural or artificial UV light to this region of the skin during the next 24 hours.

12. The patient is to return to the phototherapy center in 24 hours.

13. The area of the phototesting should be identified by the markings at the different dosage sites.

14. Identifiable erythema within the margins of the phototesting port is considered a positive reading.

15. If bright red erythema develops or blistering occurs at the site of any of the phototesting sites, then topical corticosteroids can be used to treat the area.

NARROWBAND ULTRAVIOLET B PHOTOTHERAPY BY SKIN TYPE

PATIENT INSTRUCTIONS

1. All patients designated for the NBUVB by skin type protocol will have the routine introduction to the PTC facility.

2. All patients designated for the NBUVB by skin type protocol will have the basic introduction to phototherapy equipment and safety procedures.

3. Reinforcement of the need for eye protection and covering of the genital area in males is required.

4. Patients are to stand in the center of the light cabinet with their arms at rest. A step stool may be used for the patients to stand on when recommended by the physician.

5. A handheld timer will be set by the phototherapy technician for each treatment session. The time will correspond to the estimated time of the treatment session duration, and the timer will either be given to the patient to have with them during the treatment session or be kept by the technician during the treatment. The time will correspond with the amount of time calculated for their dose of NBUVB for that treatment.

6. Instruct patients to come out of the light box when the lights have gone out or within 10 seconds of the alarm of the safety (handheld) timer. Inform patients that the light-box doors are not locked and demonstrate their operation.

7. The list of current medications will be placed in the patient's chart and reviewed by the phototherapist. Questions concerning current medications will be addressed by the attending physician.

8. All patients will be told of the possible complications of NBUVB phototherapy specifically including

    a. Sunburn reaction
    b. Corneal burn if the eyes are unprotected
    c. Photoallergic dermatitis (including drug reaction)
    d. Freckling of the skin
    e. Aging of the skin
    f. Possible increase in risk of skin cancers

9. Patients will be told that additional unprotected sun exposure should be avoided on the days they receive NBUVB. Sunblock (SPF 15) should be used on any sun-exposed areas for the remainder of that day.

10. All patients will be given the brochure on UVB phototherapy from the National Psoriasis Foundation.

PROTOCOL

1. Obtain a signed consent form after the patient has been given the tour of the PTC and basic phototherapy education concerning NBUVB phototherapy. The patient should be given time for questions.

2. Determine the skin type of the individual. See Appendix.

3. Have the patient undress completely and apply mineral oil to areas of psoriasis prior to the treatment. Male patients should wear an athletic supporter unless otherwise directed or permitted by the attending physician.

4. Eye protection in the form of UV goggles must be worn by all patients when inside the phototherapy unit.

5. The irradiance (mW/cm^2) of the NBUVB light inside the unit should be recorded on a once-a-month basis using the standard method of the manufacturer of the phototherapy unit. Record this irradiance on the phototherapy record sheet or keep an irradiance logbook for the equipment used in patient care.

6. The initial NBUVB dose (mJ/cm^2) will be based on the patient's skin type determination. The skin type will be included on the phototherapy treatment record.

Skin Type	Initial NBUVB Dose (mJ/cm^2)
Type I	300
Type II	300
Type III	500
Type IV	500
Type V	800
Type VI	800

7. The manual method for calculation of the time (seconds) to set the NBUVB control panel to deliver the dose from #6 is the following equation: (The measurement of the irradiance can be obtained from the logbook kept on a weekly basis.)

    Time (seconds) = Dose (mJ/cm^2) ÷ Irradiance (mW/cm^2)

8. The duration of a treatment or total dose of NBUVB to be delivered can often be calculated by the UV light unit by following the manufacturer's instructions in the operations manual and inputting the correct information on the control panel prior to the delivery of the treatment.

9. Set the time (or dose) on the control panel of the UV light unit and on the additional safety timer kept in the light unit or by the technician. In some phototherapy units, the session duration is dependent on the dose measured by an internal photometer, and the time must be estimated by the technician.

10. Verify that the UV light unit is set on NBUVB.

11. Turn on the fan and have the patient stand in the center of the UV light unit with their arms at rest. Double-check that they are wearing UV goggles as eye protection.

12. Instruct the patient to come out of the UV light box when the lights go out or if they become uncomfortable during the treatment either from burning or stinging of the skin. Inform the patient that the light-box doors are not locked.

13. Start the treatment.

SUBSEQUENT TREATMENTS

14. The frequency of NBUVB using MED light treatments for the diagnosis of psoriasis is 3–4 times a week unless otherwise ordered by a physician. If less than 3 times a week has been ordered by a physician, then special instructions for the advancement of the dose of NBUVB light must accompany the request.

15. On subsequent visits, the patient will be asked about redness, light pink color, and tenderness of the skin the previous night, and this information will be put into the phototherapy record.

16. If the skin is a light pink color, the phototherapist should keep the dose the same as the previously delivered treatment dose.

17. If the skin is red, the phototherapy technician will ask that the patient be seen by the attending physician who will make the decision for adjustment in the NBUVB treatment.

18. Increase the dose (mJ/cm^2) of the NBUVB light by the amount as follows, and add it to the previous dose delivered to the patient if the treatment has been within 3 days:

Skin Type	Amount of NBUVB Increase (mJ/cm^2)
Type I	100
Type II	100
Type III	125
Type IV	125
Type V	150
Type VI	150

19. Do not exceed the maximum dose indicated in the following table unless otherwise ordered by the physician:

Skin Type	Maximum NBUVB Dose (mJ/cm^2)
Type I	2000
Type II	2000
Type III	3000
Type IV	3000
Type V	5000
Type VI	5000

20. For subsequent treatments, here are the corresponding steps if the following time between treatments have been observed:

4–7 days	Keep the dose the same.
1–2 weeks	Decrease the dose by 25%.
2–4 weeks	Decrease the dose by 50%.
More than 4 weeks	Start over.

21. Follow steps 7–13 previously.

MAINTENANCE THERAPY FOR NBUVB

Once there has been acceptable improvement in the severity of the psoriasis, patients may be kept on intermittent treatments as a maintenance therapy. There is great variability in selection of the optimal frequency and dose of NBUVB needed to keep an acceptable control of psoriasis. The following general guidelines may be used:

If psoriasis has cleared (>75%), consider the following guidelines:

Once a week treatments for 4 weeks	Keep the dose the same.
Once every 2 weeks	Decrease the dose by 25%.

The activity of the underlying psoriatic condition may require long-term maintenance therapy, especially during the winter months or in locations of northern latitudes. If there has been an acceptable response (75%–100% clearance), then maintenance therapy at once every 2 weeks can be continued to keep the activity of the psoriasis under control in many patients. Long-term therapy whether in the form of combination therapy or systemic therapy would need to be discussed between the patient and physician.

SYSTEMIC PSORALEN PLUS ULTRAVIOLET A

PATIENT INSTRUCTIONS

1. All patients designated for psoralen plus ultraviolet A (PUVA) will have the routine introduction to the PTC facility.

2. All patients designated for PUVA will have the basic introduction to phototherapy equipment and safety procedures.

3. Reinforcement of the need for eye protection for all patients and covering of the genital area in males is required.

4. Patients receiving systemic PUVA will be instructed to take Oxsoralen Ultra® tablets in the dose prescribed by their physician 1 hour prior to the estimated time of their arrival at the PTC. The treatment will be given between 1 hour 15 minutes and 1 hour 45 minutes after the ingestion of the medication.

5. All patients ingesting Oxsoralen Ultra must wear protective UV blocking glasses when outside, riding in a car, or next to a window from the time they take the medication and for the next 18–24 hours during daylight.

6. Patients are to stand in the center of the light cabinet with their arms at rest. A step stool may be used for the patient to stand on when recommended by the physician.

7. A handheld timer will be set by the phototherapy technician for each treatment session. The time will correspond to the estimated time of the treatment session duration, and the timer will either be given to the patients to have with them during the treatment session or be kept by the technician during the treatment. The time will correspond with the amount of time calculated for their dose of UVA for that treatment.

8. Instruct patients to come out of the light box when the lights have gone out or within 10 seconds of the alarm of the safety (handheld) timer. Inform patients that the light-box doors are not locked and demonstrate their operation.

9. The list of current medications will be placed in the patient's chart and reviewed by the phototherapist. Questions concerning the current medications will be addressed by the attending physician.

10. All patients will be told of the possible complications of PUVA phototherapy specifically including

    a. Sunburn reaction
    b. Corneal burn if the eyes are unprotected
    c. Cataract formation if the eyes are unprotected

    d.   Photoallergic dermatitis (including drug reaction)
    e.   Freckling of the skin
    f.   Aging of the skin
    g.   Increase in risk of skin cancers including melanoma

11. Patients will be told that additional unprotected sun exposure should be avoided on the days they receive PUVA. Wide-spectrum sunblock (UVA/B) should be used on any sun-exposed areas for the remainder of that day.

12. All patients will be given the brochure on PUVA phototherapy from the National Psoriasis Foundation.

PROTOCOL

1. Obtain a signed consent form (see page 147) after the patient has been given the tour of the PTC and basic phototherapy education concerning PUVA phototherapy (see page 151). The patient should be given time for questions.

2. Oxsoralen Ultra (8-methoxypsoralen [8-MOP]) is to be ingested by the patient at least 1 hour prior to arrival at the PTC. Treatments may be given anytime between 1 hour 15 minutes and 1 hour 45 minutes after ingestion.

3. Dosage of the Oxsoralen Ultra tablets is dependent on the orders of the attending physician and may vary from patient to patient. The standard dosage is 0.5–0.6 mg/kg.

4. Ask the patient at what time they ingested their medication and how many pills they ingested.

5. Have the patient undress completely unless otherwise ordered by the physician. Male patients should wear an athletic supporter unless otherwise directed or permitted by the attending physician. Patients may apply mineral oil on the plaques of psoriasis prior to the delivery of UVA light, but this is not mandatory for PUVA.

6. Eye protection in the form of UV goggles must be worn by all patients when inside the phototherapy unit.

7. The irradiance (mW/cm^2) of the UVA light inside the unit should be recorded on a once-a-month basis using the standard method of the manufacturer of the phototherapy unit. Record this irradiance on the phototherapy record sheet or keep an irradiance logbook for the equipment used in patient care.

8. Determine the initial PUVA dose (J/cm^2) according to the patient's skin type as classified by the physician. See Appendix for definitions of skin types.

Skin Type	Initial UVA Dose (J/cm^2)
Type I	1
Type II	1
Type III	2
Type IV	2
Type V	4
Type VI	4

9. The manual method for calculation of the time (seconds) to set the UVA control panel to deliver the dose from #8 is the following equation: (The measurement of the irradiance can be obtained from the logbook kept on a weekly basis.)

$$\text{Time (seconds)} = \text{Dose } (mJ/cm^2) \div \text{Irradiance } (mW/cm^2)$$

10. The duration of a treatment or total dose of UVA to be delivered can often be calculated by the UV light unit by following the manufacturer's instructions in the operations manual and inputting the correct information on the control panel prior to the delivery of the treatment.

11. Set the time (or dose) on the control panel of the UV light unit and on the additional safety timer kept in the light unit or by the technician. In some phototherapy units, the session duration is dependent on the dose measured by an internal photometer, and the time must be estimated by the technician.

12. Verify that the UV light unit is set on UVA.

13. Turn on the fan and have the patient stand in the center of the UV light unit with their arms at rest. Double-check that they are wearing UV goggles as eye protection.

14. Instruct the patient to come out of the UV light box when the lights go out or if they become uncomfortable during the treatment either from burning or stinging of the skin. Inform the patient that the light-box doors are not locked.

15. Start the treatment.

16. Some patients may receive localized UV light therapy to the legs or trunk as ordered by the physician. See protocol for localized UVA.

17. An ophthalmology examination should be performed at the initiation of treatment and every 6 months during PUVA therapy.

18. Laboratory monitoring is done at baseline and every 6 months as necessary.

SUBSEQUENT TREATMENTS

19. The frequency of PUVA treatments for the diagnosis of psoriasis is 2 or 3 times a week unless otherwise ordered by a physician. If more than 3 times a week has been ordered, then special instructions as to the advancement of the dose of UVA light must accompany the request.

20. On subsequent visits, the patient will be asked about redness, light pink color, and tenderness of the skin the previous night, and this information will be put into the phototherapy record. The patient will also be asked at what time they took the psoralen tablets.

21. If the skin is red, the phototherapist will ask that the patient be seen by the attending physician who will make the decision for adjustment in the treatment for that day. If the skin is a light pink color, the phototherapist should keep the dose the same as the previously delivered treatment dose.

22. Increase the dose (J/cm^2) of the UVA light by the amount as follows, and add it to the previous dose delivered to the patient if the treatment has been within 3 days:

Skin Type	Amount of UVA Increase (J/cm^2)
Type I	0.5
Type II	1.0
Type III	1.0
Type IV	1.0
Type V	1.0
Type VI	1.0

23. If subsequent treatments occur at intervals longer than 3 days, the following guidelines will be used:

4–7 days	Keep the dose the same
1–2 weeks	Decrease dose by 25%
2–3 weeks	Decrease dose by 50%
3–4 weeks	Decrease dose by 75%
More than 4 weeks	Start over

24. Follow steps 4–15 previously.

MAINTENANCE THERAPY FOR PUVA

Once there has been acceptable improvement in the severity of the psoriasis, patients may be kept on intermittent treatments as a maintenance therapy. There is great variability in selection of the optimal frequency and dose of PUVA needed to keep an acceptable control of psoriasis. The following general guidelines may be used:

If psoriasis has cleared (>75%), the following guidelines can be considered:

Once a week treatment for 4 weeks	Keep the dose the same.
Once every 2 weeks long term	Decrease the dose by 25% and hold.
Once every 2–4 weeks long term	Decrease the dose by 25% and hold.

The activity of the underlying psoriatic condition may require long-term maintenance therapy, especially during the winter months or in locations of northern latitudes. If there has been an acceptable response (75%–100% clearance), then maintenance therapy at once every 2–4 weeks can be continued to keep the activity of the psoriasis under control in many patients. Long-term therapy, whether in the form of combination therapy or systemic therapy, would need to be discussed between the patient and physician.

TOPICAL PSORALEN PLUS ULTRAVIOLET A

There are two main delivery systems for topical PUVA. The psoralen molecule can either be suspended in an aqueous solution or in a lotion base for application to specific sites of the body. The most frequent and practical use of bath PUVA is for the hands and feet and is used for localized treatment of psoriasis or resistant hand and foot eczematous dermatitis. 8-MOP, the molecule most commonly used in North America, is less photosensitizing than trimethylpsoralen. 8-MOP can also be used for bath PUVA and has been used for decades with excellent results.

PATIENT INSTRUCTIONS FOR PSORALEN BATH (OR SOAK) PLUS ULTRAVIOLET A

1. All patients designated for bath PUVA will have the routine introduction to the PTC facility.

2. All patients designated for bath PUVA will have the basic introduction to phototherapy equipment and safety procedures.

3. Reinforcement of the need for eye protection for all patients and covering of the genital area in males is required if total body PUVA is to be given.

4. Patients receiving bath PUVA will be instructed to soak the areas to be treated for 15 minutes immediately preceding the delivery of the UVA light.

5. All patients receiving bath PUVA must wear protective UV blocking glasses when receiving the UVA light, riding in a car, or next to a window from the time they complete the soak and for the next 1–2 hours during daylight.

6. A handheld timer, set by the phototherapy technician, will be given to the patient to have with them during each phototherapy session. The time will correspond with the amount of time calculated for their dose of UVA for that treatment.

7. Instruct patients to complete the treatment session when the lights have gone out or within 10 seconds of the alarm of the safety (handheld) timer.

8. The list of current medications will be placed in the patient's chart and reviewed by the phototherapist. Questions concerning the current medications will be addressed by the attending physician.

9. All patients will be told of the possible complications of bath PUVA phototherapy specifically including

    a. Sunburn reaction
    b. Corneal burn if the eyes are unprotected

        c.   Cataract formation if the eyes are unprotected
        d.   Photoallergic dermatitis (including drug reaction)
        e.   Freckling of the skin
        f.   Aging of the skin
        g.   Increase in risk of skin cancers including melanoma

10.   Patients will be told that additional sunbathing should be avoided on the days they receive PUVA. Sunblock (UVA/B) should be used on any sun-exposed areas for the remainder of that day.

11.   All patients will be given the brochure on PUVA phototherapy from the National Psoriasis Foundation.

PROTOCOL

1. Obtain a signed consent form after the patient has been given the tour of the PTC and basic phototherapy education concerning PUVA phototherapy. The patient should be given time for questions.

2. Dilute 1 mL of 8-MOP lotion (10 mg/mL standard solution) in 2 L of warm water in a basin, or dilute 10 mL 0.1 mg/mL trioxsalen (trimethylpsoralen in 95% ethyl alcohol) in 2 L of warm water which must be agitated during soaking.

3. Soak the patient's hands and/or feet for 15 minutes. Set a handheld timer to be kept with the patient during the soaking procedure. Dry the skin by patting the surface with a dry towel. Wrap the wrist with multiple layers of cloth to provide protection from UVA light (*optional*). Other methods may be used to protect the skin at the wrist.

4. The irradiance (mW/cm^2) of the UVA light unit should be recorded on a once-a-month basis using the standard method of the manufacturer of the phototherapy unit. Record this irradiance on the phototherapy record sheet or keep an irradiance logbook for the equipment used in patient care.

5. The manual method for calculation of the time (seconds) to set the UV control panel to deliver the dose from #10 is the following equation: (The measurement of the irradiance can be obtained from the logbook kept on a weekly basis.)

$$\text{Time (seconds)} = \text{Dose (mJ/cm}^2) \div \text{Irradiance (mW/cm}^2)$$

6. The duration of a treatment or total dose of UV light to be delivered can often be calculated by the UV light unit by following the manufacturer's instructions in the operations manual and inputting the correct information on the control panel prior to the delivery of the treatment.

7. Set the time (or dose) on the control panel of the UV light unit and on the additional safety timer kept in the light unit or by the technician. In some phototherapy units, the session duration is dependent on the dose measured by an internal photometer, and the time must be estimated by the technician.

8. Verify that the UV light unit is set on UVA.

9. Have the patient put on protective glasses during the phototherapy treatment session and for 1 hour after treatment.

10. Begin the treatment at 0.5 J/cm^2 UVA for all skin types.

11. After the UVA treatment is given, the patient must thoroughly wash his hands and/or feet to remove any medication residue on the surface of the skin. Sunblock (UVA/B) is provided for the patient to apply as a precautionary measure to avoid additional UVA exposure that day.

12. Instruct the patient to avoid excessive sunlight for the remainder of the day. A burn may not show up until 48 hours after treatment. Treatments are not usually given on 2 consecutive days. This allows the nurse to observe accurately for erythema.

SUBSEQUENT TREATMENTS

13. Increase by 0.5 J/cm^2 every treatment as tolerated. Consult the attending physician if burning has occurred.

14. Do not exceed a dose of 2.5 J/cm^2 for a treatment unless instructed by the physician.

15. The frequency of bath PUVA treatments for the diagnosis of psoriasis is 2 or 3 times a week unless otherwise ordered by a physician. If more than 3 times a week has been ordered, then special instructions as to the advancement of the dose of UVA light must accompany the request.

16. If the skin is red or painful, the phototherapist will ask that the patient be seen by the attending physician who will make the decision for adjustment in the treatment for that day. If the skin is a light pink color, the phototherapist should keep the dose the same as the previously delivered treatment dose.

17. If subsequent treatments occur at intervals longer than 3 days, the following guidelines will be used:

3–7 days	Keep the dose the same.
1–2 weeks	Decrease the dose by 50%.
3 weeks	Start over.

18. Follow steps 2–12 previously.

PATIENT INSTRUCTIONS FOR PSORALEN PAINT (LOTION) PLUS ULTRAVIOLET A

1. All patients designated for paint PUVA will have the routine introduction to the PTC facility.

2. All patients designated for paint PUVA will have the basic introduction to phototherapy equipment and safety procedures.

3. Reinforcement of the need for eye protection for all patients and covering of the genital area in males is required if total body PUVA is to be given.

4. Patients receiving paint PUVA will be instructed to apply the psoralen lotion with a cotton-tipped applicator to the areas to be treated for 30 minutes immediately preceding the delivery of the UVA light. This area is to be protected or covered with protective fabric if application of the psoralen was done outside the confines of the treatment center.

5. All patients receiving paint PUVA must wear protective clothing or sunblock containing both UVA and UVB sunscreen after washing the treated areas following the delivery of UVA light.

6. A handheld timer, set by the phototherapy technician, will be given to the patient to have with them during each phototherapy session. The time will correspond with the amount of time calculated for their dose of UVA for that treatment.

7. Instruct patients to complete the treatment session when the lights have gone out or within 10 seconds of the alarm of the safety (handheld) timer.

8. A list of current medications will be placed in the patient's chart and reviewed by the phototherapist. Questions concerning the current medications will be addressed by the attending physician.

9. All patients will be told of the possible complications of paint PUVA phototherapy specifically including

   a. Sunburn reaction
   b. Corneal burn if the eyes are unprotected
   c. Cataract formation if the eyes are unprotected
   d. Photoallergic dermatitis (including drug reaction)
   e. Freckling of the skin
   f. Aging of the skin
   g. Increase in risk of skin cancers including melanoma

10. Patients will be told that additional sun exposure should be avoided on the days they receive paint PUVA. The patients should be told that UVA light is transmitted through window and auto glass.

11. All patients will be given the brochure on PUVA phototherapy from the National Psoriasis Foundation.

PROTOCOL

1. Obtain a signed consent form after the patient has been given the tour of the PTC and basic phototherapy education concerning PUVA phototherapy. The patient should be given time for questions.

2. A lotion containing 0.01% of 8-MOP should be prescribed to the patient for their use. The compounding of this lotion should be carried out by a pharmacist. The 8-MOP may also be prepared in an ointment base using Aquaphor or a Vaseline base. The concentration for the ointment-based psoralen preparation is 0.1% of 8-MOP.

3. Apply the psoralen lotion to the involved areas with a cotton-tipped applicator. Only apply the psoralen to the sites to be treated. This is best done in the treatment center with the aid of a technician, especially in the case of hard-to-reach areas. However, the lotion may be applied by the patient prior to the time of the scheduled treatment with UVA. The duration of the pretreatment with the topical psoralen should be 30 minutes. The delivery of the dose of UVA light should follow the 30-minute pretreatment period. Uninvolved areas adjacent to the treated sites can be wrapped with multiple layers of cloth to provide protection from UVA light (*optional*).

4. The initial dose of UVA for paint PUVA is 0.5 J/cm^2 for all skin types.

5. The irradiance (mW/cm^2) of the UVA light unit should be recorded on a once-a-month basis using the standard method of the manufacturer of the phototherapy unit. Record this irradiance on the phototherapy record sheet or keep an irradiance logbook for the equipment used in patient care.

6. The manual method for calculation of the time (seconds) to set the UV control panel to deliver the dose from #4 is the following equation: (The measurement of the irradiance can be obtained from the logbook kept on a weekly basis.)

$$\text{Time (seconds)} = \text{Dose (mJ/cm}^2) \div \text{Irradiance (mW/cm}^2)$$

7. The duration of a treatment or total dose of UV light to be delivered can often be calculated by the UV light unit by following the manufacturer's instructions in the operations manual and inputting the correct information on the control panel prior to the delivery of the treatment.

8. Set the time (or dose) on the control panel of the UV light unit and on the additional safety timer kept in the light unit or by the technician. In some phototherapy units, the session duration is dependent on the dose measured by an internal photometer, and the time must be estimated by the technician.

9. Verify that the UV light unit is set on UVA.

10. Have the patient put on protective glasses during the phototherapy treatment session.

11. Start the treatment.

12. After the UVA treatment is given, the patient must thoroughly wash the treated areas to remove any medication residue on the surface of the skin. Sunblock (UVA/B) is provided for the patient to apply as a precautionary measure to avoid additional UV exposure that day.

13. Instruct the patient to avoid excessive sunlight the remainder of the day. A burn may not show up until 48 hours after treatment. Treatments are not usually given on 2 consecutive days. This allows the nurse to observe accurately for erythema.

14. Advise the patient that areas around the psoriasis may become darker in color as treatments progress.

15. Each patient should be seen by the attending physician 2 weeks after the first treatment, and then every 2–4 weeks during treatment. The patient should be seen immediately by a physician if any burning, blistering, or pain at treatment sites occurs.

SUBSEQUENT TREATMENTS

16. Increase the dose by 0.5 J/cm^2 every treatment as tolerated up to 4 J/cm^2. Consult the attending physician if burning has occurred. Higher doses of UVA must be ordered by the physician.

17. The frequency of paint PUVA treatments for the diagnosis of psoriasis is 2 times a week unless otherwise ordered by a physician. If more than 2 times a week has been ordered, then special instructions as to the advancement of the dose of UVA light must accompany the request.

18. If the skin is red the phototherapist will contact the attending physician who will make the decision for adjustment in the treatment for that day. If the skin is a light pink color, the phototherapist should keep the dose the same as the previously delivered treatment dose.

19. If subsequent treatments occur at intervals longer than 3 days, the following guidelines will be used:

4–7 days	Keep the dose the same.
1–2 weeks	Decrease the dose by 50%.
More than 3 weeks	Start over.

20. Follow steps 3–15 previously.

RETINOID PLUS ULTRAVIOLET B PHOTOTHERAPY

PATIENT INSTRUCTIONS

1. All patients designated for the retinoid plus UVB (ReUVB) protocol will have the routine introduction to the PTC facility.

2. All patients designated for the ReUVB protocol will have the basic introduction to phototherapy equipment and safety procedures.

3. Reinforcement of the need for eye protection and covering of the genital area in males is required.

4. All patients with the diagnosis of psoriasis will be told to apply mineral oil to the involved areas of the skin prior to the delivery of UVB.

5. Patients are to stand in the center of the light cabinet with their arms at rest. A step stool may be used for the patients to stand on when recommended by the physician.

6. A handheld timer will be set by the phototherapy technician for each treatment session. The time will correspond to the estimated time of the treatment session duration, and the timer will either be given to the patient to have with them during the treatment session or be kept by the technician during the treatment. The time will correspond with the amount of time calculated for their dose of UVB for that treatment.

7. Instruct patients to come out of the light box when the lights have gone out or within 10 seconds of the alarm of the safety (handheld) timer. Inform patients that the light-box doors are not locked and demonstrate their operation.

8. The list of current medications will be placed in the patient's chart and reviewed by the phototherapist. Questions concerning current medications will be addressed by the attending physician.

9. All patients will be told of the possible complications of UVB phototherapy specifically including

    a. Sunburn reaction
    b. Corneal burn if the eyes are unprotected
    c. Photoallergic dermatitis (including drug reaction)
    d. Freckling of the skin
    e. Aging of the skin
    f. Possible increase in risk of skin cancers

10. Patients will be told that additional unprotected sun exposure should be avoided on the days they receive UVB. Sunblock (SPF 15) should be used on any sun-exposed areas for the remainder of that day.

11. All patients will be given the brochure on UVB phototherapy and retinoid therapy from the National Psoriasis Foundation.

PROTOCOL

The dose of the retinoid used, either acitretin (Soriatane®), 13-*cis*-retinoic acid, or other retinoids approved in the future for treatment of psoriasis will be determined by the physician. Initiation of the retinoid therapy should be done 1–2 weeks prior to the start of the UVB treatments. The use of retinoid therapy for psoriasis, its effects and potential side effects, will be discussed with the patient. The usual starting dose of Soriatane for combination treatment is 25 mg/day but can be adjusted according to other factors at the time of the evaluation by the physician. The dose of the retinoid would then be adjusted during the course of therapy according to the physician's orders dependent upon the clinical response with a decrease in the dose of the retinoid usually within the first 2 months of UV therapy. Ask the patient what dose they are currently taking and document the dose on the phototherapy flow sheet.

If the systemic retinoid is started after the patient has already undergone induction of UVB therapy, then the dose of the UVB should be reduced by 50% of the dose used prior to the initiation of the retinoid. The dose of UVB should not be increased for 2 weeks after the introduction of the systemic retinoid.

1. Obtain a signed consent form after the patient has been given the tour of the PTC and basic phototherapy education concerning ReUVB phototherapy. The patient should be given time for questions.

2. Have the patient undress completely. Male patients should wear an athletic supporter unless otherwise directed or permitted by the attending physician. Patients will apply mineral oil on the plaques of psoriasis prior to the delivery of UV light.

3. Eye protection in the form of UV goggles must be worn by all patients when inside the phototherapy unit.

4. The irradiance (mW/cm^2) of the UVB light inside the unit should be recorded on a once-a-month basis using the standard method of the manufacturer of the phototherapy unit. Record this irradiance on the phototherapy record sheet or keep an irradiance logbook for the equipment used in patient care.

5. Determine the initial UVB dose (mJ/cm^2) according to the patient's skin type as classified by the physician. See Appendix for definitions of skin types.

Skin Type	Initial UVB Dose (mJ/cm^2)
Type I	20
Type II	25
Type III	30
Type IV	40
Type V	50
Type VI	60

6. The manual method for calculation of the time (seconds) to set the UVB control panel to deliver the dose from #5 is the following equation: (The measurement of the irradiance can be obtained from the logbook kept on a weekly basis.)

$$\text{Time (seconds)} = \text{Dose (mJ/cm}^2) \div \text{Irradiance (mW/cm}^2)$$

7. The duration of a treatment or total dose of UVB to be delivered can often be calculated by the UV light unit by following the manufacturer's instructions in the operations manual and inputting the correct information on the control panel prior to the delivery of the treatment.

8. Set the time (or dose) on the control panel of the UV light unit and on the additional safety timer kept in the light unit or by the technician. In some phototherapy units, the session duration is dependent on the dose measured by an internal photometer, and the time must be estimated by the technician.

9. Verify that the UV light unit is set on UVB.

10. Turn on the fan and have the patient stand in the center of the UV light unit with their arms at rest. Double-check that they are wearing UV goggles as eye protection.

11. Instruct the patient to come out of the UV light box when the lights go out or if they become uncomfortable during the treatment either from burning or stinging of the skin. Inform the patient that the light-box doors are not locked.

12. Start the treatment.

SUBSEQUENT TREATMENTS

13. The frequency of ReUVB light treatments for the diagnosis of psoriasis is 3–5 times a week unless otherwise ordered by a physician. If less than 3 times a week has been ordered by a physician, then special instructions for the advancement of the dose of UVB light must accompany the request.

14. On subsequent visits, the patient will be asked about redness and tenderness of the skin the previous night, and this information will be put into the phototherapy record.

15. If the skin is a light pink color, the phototherapist should keep the dose the same as the previously delivered treatment dose.

16. If the skin is red, the phototherapy technician will ask that the patient be seen by the attending physician who will make the decision for adjustment in the UVB treatment.

17. Increase the dose (mJ/cm^2) of the UVB light by the amount as follows, and add it to the previous dose delivered to the patient if the treatment has been within 3 days:

Skin Type	Amount of UVB Increase (mJ/cm^2)
Type I	5
Type II	10
Type III	15
Type IV	20
Type V	25
Type VI	30

18. For subsequent treatments, here are the corresponding steps if the following time between treatments have been observed:

4–7 days	Keep the dose the same.
1–2 weeks	Decrease the dose by 25%.
2–4 weeks	Decrease the dose by 50%.
More than 4 weeks	Start over.

19. Follow steps 6–12 previously.

RETINOID PLUS NARROWBAND ULTRAVIOLET B

PATIENT INSTRUCTIONS

1. The combination of a systemic retinoid plus NBUVB (ReNBUVB) is best done using the NBUVB by MED protocol. This is especially important when the treatment plan is to start with the retinoid therapy for 1–2 weeks then initiate the NBUVB treatments. Obtaining the MED at that time will give a much more accurate and, thus, effective dose of NBUVB for the initiation of NBUVB and will help avoid phototoxic reactions from the treatments.

2. All patients designated for the ReNBUVB protocol will have the routine introduction to the PTC facility.

3. All patients designated for the ReNBUVB protocol will have the basic introduction to phototherapy equipment and safety procedures.

4. Reinforcement of the need for eye protection and covering of the genital area in males is required.

5. Patients are to stand in the center of the light cabinet with their arms at rest. A step stool may be used for the patients to stand on when recommended by the physician.

6. A handheld timer will be set by the phototherapy technician for each treatment session. The time will correspond to the estimated time of the treatment session duration, and the timer will either be given to the patients to have with them during the treatment session or be kept by the technician during the treatment. The time will correspond with the amount of time calculated for their dose of NBUVB for that treatment.

7. Instruct patients to come out of the light box when the lights have gone out or within 10 seconds of the alarm of the safety (handheld) timer. Inform patients that the light-box doors are not locked and demonstrate their operation.

8. The list of current medications will be placed in the patient's chart and reviewed by the phototherapist. Questions concerning current medications will be addressed by the attending physician.

9. All patients will be told of the possible complications of NBUVB photo-therapy specifically including

    a.   Sunburn reaction
    b.   Corneal burn if the eyes are unprotected
    c.   Photoallergic dermatitis (including drug reaction)
    d.   Freckling of the skin
    e.   Aging of the skin
    f.   Possible increase in risk of skin cancers

10. Patients will be told that additional unprotected sun exposure should be avoided on the days they receive NBUVB. Sunblock (SPF 15) should be used on any sun-exposed areas for the remainder of that day.

11. All patients will be given the brochure on UVB phototherapy and retinoid therapy from the National Psoriasis Foundation.

PROTOCOL

The dose of the retinoid used, either acitretin (Soriatane), 13-*cis*-retinoic acid or other retinoids approved in the future for treatment of psoriasis, will be determined by the physician. Initiation of the retinoid therapy should be done 1–2 weeks prior to the start of NBUVB treatments. The use of retinoid therapy for psoriasis, its effects and potential side effects will be discussed with the patient. The usual starting dose of Soriatane for the combination treatment is 25 mg/day but can be adjusted according to other factors at the time of the evaluation by the physician. The dose of the retinoid would then be adjusted during the course of therapy according to the physician's orders dependent upon the clinical response with a decrease in the dose of the retinoid usually within the first 2 months of UV therapy. Ask the patient what dose they are currently taking and document the dose on the phototherapy flow sheet.

If the systemic retinoid is started after the patient has already undergone induction of NBUVB therapy, then the dose of the NBUVB should be reduced by 50% of the dose used prior to the initiation of the retinoid. The dose of NBUVB should not be increased for 2 weeks after the introduction of the systemic retinoid.

1. Obtain a signed consent form after the patient has been given the tour of the PTC and basic phototherapy education concerning NBUVB phototherapy. The patient should be given time for questions.

2. One to two weeks after the initiation of retinoid therapy, obtain an MED from the lower lumbar or sacral area using the standard procedure. See the section "Procedure for Determination of the MED for NBUVB."

3. Have the patient undress completely. Male patients should wear an athletic supporter unless otherwise directed or permitted by the attending physician.

4. Eye protection in the form of UV goggles must be worn by all patients when inside the phototherapy unit.

5. The irradiance (mW/cm^2) of the NBUVB light inside the unit should be recorded on a once-a-month basis using the standard method of the manufacturer of the phototherapy unit. Record this irradiance on the phototherapy record sheet or keep an irradiance logbook for the equipment used in patient care.

6. The initial NBUVB dose (mJ/cm^2) will be based on the patient's MED determination at 24 hours from the delivery of the test doses. The MED will be included in the phototherapy treatment record.

Initial NBUVB = 50% of the MED

(If the patient's MED is higher than the highest test dose of NBUVB delivered in the MED determination testing, then a dose of 50% of the highest test site will be used as the initial dose.)

7. The manual method for calculation of the time (seconds) to set the NBUVB control panel to deliver the dose from #6 is the following equation: (The measurement of the irradiance can be obtained from the logbook kept on a weekly basis.)

$$\text{Time (seconds)} = \text{Dose (mJ/cm}^2) \div \text{Irradiance (mW/cm}^2)$$

8. The duration of a treatment or total dose of NBUVB to be delivered can often be calculated by the UV light unit by following the manufacturer's instructions in the operations manual and inputting the correct information on the control panel prior to the delivery of the treatment.

9. Set the time (or dose) on the control panel of the UV light unit and on the additional safety timer kept in the light unit or by the technician. In some phototherapy units, the session duration is dependent on the dose measured by an internal photometer, and the time must be estimated by the technician.

10. Verify that the UV light unit is set on NBUVB.

11. Turn on the fan and have the patient stand in the center of the UV light unit with their arms at rest. Double-check that they are wearing UV goggles as eye protection.

12. Instruct the patient to come out of the UV light box when the lights go out or if they become uncomfortable during the treatment either from burning or stinging of the skin. Inform the patient that the light-box doors are not locked.

13. Start the treatment.

SUBSEQUENT TREATMENTS

14. The frequency of NBUVB using MED light treatments for the diagnosis of psoriasis is 3 times a week unless otherwise ordered by a physician. If less than 3 times a week has been ordered by a physician, then special instructions for the advancement of the dose of NBUVB light must accompany the request.

15. On subsequent visits, the patient will be asked about redness, light pink color, and tenderness of the skin the previous night, and this information will be put into the phototherapy record.

16. If the skin is red, the phototherapy technician will ask that the patient be seen by the attending physician who will make the decision for adjustment in the NBUVB treatment. If the skin is a light pink color, the phototherapist should keep the dose the same as the previously delivered treatment dose.

17. Increase the dose (mJ/cm^2) of the NBUVB light by the following amount, and add it to the previous dose delivered to the patient if the treatment has been within 3 days:

Treatments 1–20	Increase by 10% of MED.
Treatments 21–X	Increase as ordered by physician.

18. Do not exceed 4 times the MED unless otherwise ordered by the physician.

19. For subsequent treatments, if the following time between treatments have been, these corresponding steps can be done:

4–7 days	Keep the dose the same.
1–2 weeks	Decrease the dose by 25%.
2–4 weeks	Decrease the dose by 50%.
More than 4 weeks	Start over.

20. Follow the aforementioned steps 7–13.

RETINOID PLUS PSORALEN PLUS ULTRAVIOLET A

1. All patients designated for retinoid plus psoralen plus ultraviolet A (RePUVA) will have the routine introduction to the PTC facility.

2. All patients designated for RePUVA will have the basic introduction to phototherapy equipment and safety procedures.

3. Reinforcement of the need for eye protection for all patients and covering of the genital area in males is required.

4. Patients receiving RePUVA will be instructed to take Oxsoralen Ultra tablets in the dose prescribed by their physician 1 hour prior to the estimated time of their arrival at the PTC. The treatment will be given between 1 hour 15 minutes and 1 hour 45 minutes after the ingestion of the medication.

5. All patients ingesting Oxsoralen Ultra must wear protective UV blocking glasses when outside, riding in a car, or next to a window from the time they take the medication and for the next 18–24 hours during daylight.

6. Patients are to stand in the center of the light cabinet with their arms at rest. A step stool may be used for the patient to stand on when recommended by the physician.

7. A handheld timer will be set by the phototherapy technician for each treatment session. The time will correspond to the estimated time of the treatment session duration, and the timer will either be given to the patients to have with them during the treatment session or be kept by the technician during the treatment. The time will correspond with the amount of time calculated for their dose of UVA for that treatment.

8. Instruct patients to come out of the light box when the lights have gone out or within 10 seconds of the alarm of the safety (handheld) timer. Inform patients that the light-box doors are not locked and demonstrate their operation.

9. The list of current medications will be placed in the patient's chart and reviewed by the phototherapist. Questions concerning the current medications will be addressed by the attending physician.

10. All patients will be told of the possible complications of RePUVA photo-therapy specifically including

    a.   Sunburn reaction
    b.   Corneal burn if the eyes are unprotected
    c.   Cataract formation if the eyes are unprotected
    d.   Photoallergic dermatitis (including drug reaction)
    e.   Freckling of the skin
    f.   Aging of the skin
    g.   Increase in risk of skin cancers including melanoma

11. Patients will be told that additional unprotected sun exposure should be avoided on the days they receive RePUVA. Wide-spectrum sunblock (UVA/UVB) should be used on any sun-exposed areas for the remainder of that day.

12. All patients will be given the brochure on PUVA phototherapy from the National Psoriasis Foundation.

PROTOCOL

The dose of the retinoid used, either acitretin (Soriatane), 13-*cis*-retinoic acid or other retinoids approved in the future for treatment of psoriasis, will be determined by the physician. Initiation of the retinoid therapy should be done 1–2 weeks prior to the start of PUVA treatments. The use of retinoid therapy for psoriasis, its effects and potential side effects, will be discussed with the patient. The usual starting dose of Soriatane for combination treatment is 25 mg/day but can be adjusted according to other factors at the time of the evaluation by the physician. The dose of the retinoid would then be adjusted during the course of therapy according to the physician's orders dependent upon the clinical response with a decrease in the dose of the retinoid usually within the first 2 months of PUVA therapy. Ask the patient what dose they are currently taking and document the dose on the phototherapy flow sheet.

If the systemic retinoid is started after the patient has already undergone induction of PUVA therapy, then the dose of PUVA should be reduced by 50% of the dose used prior to the initiation of the retinoid. The dose of UVA should not be increased for 2 weeks after the introduction of the systemic retinoid.

1. Obtain a signed consent form after the patient has been given the tour of the PTC and basic phototherapy education concerning PUVA phototherapy. The patient should be given time for questions.

2. Oxsoralen Ultra (8-MOP) is to be ingested by the patient at least 1 hour prior to arrival at PTC. Treatments may be given anytime between 1 hour 15 minutes and 1 hour 45 minutes after ingestion.

3. Dosage of the Oxsoralen Ultra tablets is dependent on the orders of the attending physician and will vary from patient to patient. The standard dosage is 0.5–0.6 mg/kg.

4. Ask the patient at what time they ingested their medication and how many pills they ingested.

5. Have the patient undress completely unless otherwise ordered by the physician. Male patients should wear an athletic supporter unless otherwise directed or permitted by the attending physician. Patients may apply mineral oil on the plaques of psoriasis prior to the delivery of UVA light, but this is not mandatory for RePUVA.

6. Eye protection in the form of UV goggles must be worn by all patients when inside the phototherapy unit.

7. The irradiance (mW/cm^2) of the UVA light inside the unit should be recorded on a once-a-month basis using the standard method of the manufacturer of the phototherapy unit. Record this irradiance on the phototherapy record sheet or keep an irradiance logbook for the equipment used in patient care.

8. Determine the initial RePUVA dose (J/cm^2) according to the patient's skin type as classified by the physician. See Appendix for definitions of skin types.

Skin Type	Initial UVA Dose (J/cm^2)
Type I	0.5
Type II	0.5
Type III	1
Type IV	1
Type V	2
Type VI	2

9. The manual method for calculation of the time (seconds) to set the UVA control panel to deliver the dose from #8 is the following equation: (The measurement of the irradiance can be obtained from the logbook kept on a weekly basis.)

$$\text{Time (seconds)} = \text{Dose (mJ/cm}^2\text{)} \div \text{Irradiance (mW/cm}^2\text{)}$$

10. The duration of a treatment or total dose of UVA to be delivered can often be calculated by the UV light unit by following the manufacturer's instructions in the operations manual and inputting the correct information on the control panel prior to the delivery of the treatment.

11. Set the time (or dose) on the control panel of the UV light unit and on the additional safety timer kept in the light unit or by the technician. In some phototherapy units, the session duration is dependent on the dose measured by an internal photometer, and the time must be estimated by the technician.

12. Verify that the UV light unit is set on UVA.

13. Turn on the fan and have the patient stand in the center of the UV light unit with their arms at rest. Double-check that they are wearing UV goggles as eye protection.

14. Instruct the patient to come out of the UV light box when the lights go out or if they become uncomfortable during the treatment either from burning or stinging of the skin. Inform the patient that the light-box doors are not locked.

15. Start the treatment.

16. Some patients may receive localized UV light therapy to the legs or trunk as ordered by the physician.

17. An ophthalmology examination should be performed initially and every 6 months during RePUVA therapy.

18. Laboratory monitoring for lipid levels and hepatic enzyme elevation is carried out at baseline, 2 weeks after the start of retinoid therapy, 4 weeks after the start of retinoid therapy, and every 1–2 months during RePUVA as necessary.

SUBSEQUENT TREATMENTS

19. The frequency of RePUVA treatments for the diagnosis of psoriasis is 2 or 3 times a week unless otherwise ordered by a physician. If more than 3 times a week has been ordered, then special instructions as to the advancement of the dose of UVA light must accompany the request.

20. On subsequent visits, the patient will be asked about redness, light pink color, and tenderness of the skin the previous night, and this information will be put into the phototherapy record. The patient will also be asked at what time they took the psoralen tablets.

21. If the skin is red, the phototherapist will ask that the patient be seen by the attending physician who will make the decision for adjustment in the treatment for that day. If the skin is a light pink color, the phototherapist should keep the dose the same as the previously delivered treatment dose.

22. Increase the dose (J/cm^2) of the UVA light by the amount as follows, and add it to the previous dose delivered to the patient if the treatment has been within 3 days:

Skin Type	Amount of UVA Increase (J/cm^2)
Type I	0.5
Type II	1.0
Type III	1.0
Type IV	1.0
Type V	1.0
Type VI	1.0

23. If subsequent treatments occur at intervals longer than 3 days, the following guidelines will be used:

3–7 days	Keep the dose the same.
1–2 weeks	Decrease the dose by 25%.
2–3 weeks	Decrease the dose by 50%.
3–4 weeks	Decrease the dose by 75%.
More than 4 weeks	Start over

24. Follow steps 4–15 previously.

GOECKERMAN TREATMENT (CRUDE COAL TAR PLUS UVB)

This is modified from the original Goeckerman method.

PATIENT INSTRUCTIONS

---

1. All patients designated for Goeckerman treatments will have the routine introduction to the PTC facility.

2. All patients designated for Goeckerman treatments will have the basic introduction to phototherapy equipment and safety procedures.

3. Reinforcement of the need for eye protection for all patients and covering of the genital area in males is required.

4. Patients should be assigned a locker for the duration of their treatment at the PTC. It is their responsibility to supply a lock.

5. All patients undergoing Goeckerman treatments should understand that at least 4 hours a day of tar under occlusion with saran wrap or with occlusive garments will be part of their treatment.

6. All patients with the diagnosis of psoriasis will be told to apply mineral oil to the involved areas of the skin prior to the delivery of UVB at the start of the day's treatment.

7. Patients are to stand in the center of the light cabinet with their arms at rest. A step stool may be used for the patients to stand on when recommended by the physician.

8. A handheld timer will be set by the phototherapy technician for each treatment session. The time will correspond to the estimated time of the treatment session duration, and the timer will either be given to the patients to have with them during the treatment session or be kept by the technician during the treatment. The time will correspond with the amount of time calculated for their dose of UVB for that treatment.

9. Instruct patients to come out of the light box when the lights have gone out or within 10 seconds of the alarm of the safety (handheld) timer. Inform patients that the light-box doors are not locked and demonstrate their operation.

10. The list of current medications will be placed in the patient's chart and reviewed by the phototherapist. Questions concerning current medications will be addressed by the attending physician.

11. All patients will be asked to apply an emollient such as Aquaphor or Vaseline petroleum to the involved areas at night and leave on overnight.

12. All patients will be told of the possible complications of Goeckerman treatments specifically including

   a. Folliculitis
   b. Tar irritation
   c. Sunburn reaction
   d. Corneal burn if the eyes are unprotected
   e. Photoallergic dermatitis (including drug reaction)
   f. Freckling of the skin
   g. Aging of the skin
   h. Possible increase in risk of skin cancers

13. Patients will be told that additional sunbathing should be avoided on the days they receive Goeckerman treatments. Sunblock (SPF 15) should be used on any sun-exposed areas for the remainder of that day.

14. All patients will be given the brochure on UVB and tar from the National Psoriasis Foundation.

PROTOCOL

1. Obtain a signed consent form after the patient has been given the tour of the PTC and basic phototherapy education concerning Goeckerman treatments. The patient should be given time for questions.

2. Have the patient undress completely. Male patients should wear an athletic supporter unless otherwise directed or permitted by the attending physician. Patients will apply mineral oil on the plaques of psoriasis prior to the delivery of UV light.

3. Eye protection in the form of UV goggles must be worn by all patients when inside the phototherapy unit.

4. The irradiance (mW/cm^2) of the UVB light inside the unit should be recorded on a once-a-month basis using the standard method of the manufacturer of the phototherapy unit. Record this irradiance on the phototherapy record sheet or keep an irradiance logbook for the equipment used in the patient care.

5. Determine the initial UVB dose (mJ/cm^2) according to the patient's skin type as classified by the physician. See Appendix for definitions of skin types.

Skin Type	Initial UVB Dose (mJ/cm^2)
Type I	20
Type II	25
Type III	30
Type IV	40
Type V	50
Type VI	60

6. The manual method for calculation of the time (seconds) to set the UVB control panel to deliver the dose from #5 is the following equation: (The measurement of the irradiance can be obtained from the logbook kept on a weekly basis.)

$$\text{Time (seconds)} = \text{Dose (mJ/cm}^2) \div \text{Irradiance (mW/cm}^2)$$

7. The duration of a treatment or total dose of UVB to be delivered can often be calculated by the UV light unit by following the manufacturer's instructions in the operations manual and inputting the correct information on the control panel prior to the delivery of the treatment.

8. Set the time (or dose) on the control panel of the UV light unit and on the additional safety timer kept in the light unit or by the technician. In some phototherapy units, the session duration is dependent on the dose measured by an internal photometer, and the time must be estimated by the technician.

9. Verify that the UV light unit is set on UVB.

10. Turn on the fan and have the patient stand in the center of the UV light unit with their arms at rest. Double-check that they are wearing UV goggles as eye protection.

11. Instruct the patient to come out of the UV light box when the lights go out or if they become uncomfortable during the treatment either from burning or stinging of the skin. Inform the patient that the light-box doors are not locked.

12. Start the treatment.

13. Some patients may receive localized UV light therapy to the legs or trunk as ordered by the physician.

14. After completion of the UVB light treatment, the patient will be brought to the treatment area for application of crude coal tar. The crude coal tar is to be applied by the nursing staff from the neck down except in the axilla, groin, and body folds. Initial concentration of coal tar to be used is 2% and may increase to 5% after the first week of therapy.

15. When application of the coal tar is completed, the patient is to be wrapped with saran wrap and this is to be secured in place. The patient is then to put on surgical scrub suits supplied by the PTC. An alternative to the wrapping with saran wrap is to use an occlusive garment that has proper fitting at the neck, wrists, and ankles. A nylon or plastic body suit designed for this purpose can be acquired commercially.

16. There is to be at least 4 hours of tar under occlusion each day of Goeckerman treatment. The usual time required is 6 hours of occlusion unless otherwise specified by the attending physician.

17. The PTC lounge is provided for patients during this time of tar under occlusion.

18. Scalp debridement therapy may be performed during the 6 hour period that the patients are at the treatment center. See protocol for scalp debridement.

19. At the end of the tar occlusion period, the patient will be given a hydrosound treatment. See protocol for hydrosound treatment. Shower facilities may be used instead of the hydrosound.

20. Goeckerman treatment patients are asked to apply a heavy emollient or Aquaphor ointment to the involved areas at night and leave on overnight.

SUBSEQUENT TREATMENTS

21. The frequency of Goeckerman treatments for the diagnosis of psoriasis is 5 times a week unless otherwise ordered by a physician. If less than 4 times a week has been ordered, then special instructions for the advancement of the dose of UVB light must accompany the request.

22. On subsequent visits, the patient will be asked about redness, light pink color, and tenderness of the skin the previous night, and this information will be put into the phototherapy record.

23. If the skin is red, the phototherapist will ask that the patient be seen by the attending physician who will make the decision for adjustment in the treatment for that day. If the skin is a light pink color, the phototherapist should keep the dose the same as the previously delivered treatment dose.

24. Increase the dose (mJ/cm^2) of the UVB light by the amount as follows, and add it to the previous dose delivered to the patient if the treatment has been within 3 days:

Skin Type	Amount of UVB Increase (mJ/cm^2)
Type I	5
Type II	10
Type III	15
Type IV	20
Type V	25
Type VI	30

25. For subsequent treatments, here are the corresponding steps if the following time between treatments have been observed:

3–7 days	Keep the dose the same.
1–2 weeks	Decrease the dose by 25%.
2–3 weeks	Decrease the dose by 50%.
3–4 weeks	Decrease the dose by 75%.
More than 4 weeks	Start over.

26. Follow steps 6–20 previously.

INGRAM TREATMENT (ANTHRALIN PLUS UVB)

This is modified from the original Ingram method.

PATIENT INSTRUCTIONS

1. All patients designated for Ingram treatment will have the routine introduction to the PTC facility.

2. All patients designated for Ingram treatment will have the basic introduction to phototherapy equipment and safety procedures.

3. Reinforcement of the need for eye protection for all patients and covering of the genital area in males is required.

4. Patients should be assigned a locker for the duration of their treatment at the PTC. It is their responsibility to supply a lock.

5. All patients undergoing Ingram treatments should understand that at least 1–2 hours of treatment with varying strengths of anthralin paste applied to their skin will be part of the treatment.

6. All patients with the diagnosis of psoriasis will be told to apply mineral oil to the involved areas of the skin prior to the delivery of UVB at the start of the day's treatment.

7. Patients are to stand in the center of the light cabinet with their arms at rest. A step stool may be used for the patients to stand on when recommended by the physician.

8. A handheld timer will be set by the phototherapy technician for each treatment session. The time will correspond to the estimated time of the treatment session duration, and the timer will either be given to the patients to have with them during the treatment session or be kept by the technician during the treatment. The time will correspond with the amount of time calculated for their dose of UVB for that treatment.

9. Instruct patients to come out of the light box when the lights have gone out or within 10 seconds of the alarm of the safety (handheld) timer. Inform patients that the light-box doors are not locked and demonstrate their operation.

10. The list of current medications will be placed in the patient's chart and reviewed by the phototherapist. Questions concerning current medications will be addressed by the attending physician.

11. All patients will be told of the possible complications of Ingram treatment specifically including

      a.   Folliculitis
      b.   Anthralin staining
      c.   Anthralin irritation
      d.   Anthralin burning
      e.   Sunburn reaction
      f.   Corneal burn if the eyes are unprotected
      g.   Photoallergic dermatitis (including drug reaction)
      h.   Freckling of the skin
      i.   Aging of the skin
      j.   Possible increase in risk of skin cancers

12. Patients will be told that additional sunbathing should be avoided on the days they receive Ingram treatments. Sunblock (SPF 15) should be used on any sun-exposed areas for the remainder of that day.

13. All patients will be given the brochure on UVB and anthralin from the National Psoriasis Foundation.

PROTOCOL

1. Obtain a signed consent form after the patient has been given the tour of the PTC and basic phototherapy education concerning Ingram treatments. The patient should be given time for questions.

2. Have the patient undress completely. Male patients should wear an athletic supporter unless otherwise directed or permitted by the attending physician. Patients will apply mineral oil on the plaques of psoriasis prior to the delivery of UV light.

3. Eye protection in the form of UV goggles must be worn by all patients when inside the phototherapy unit.

4. The irradiance (mW/cm^2) of the UVB light inside the unit should be recorded on a once-a-month basis using the standard method of the manufacturer of the phototherapy unit. Record this irradiance on the phototherapy record sheet or keep an irradiance logbook for the equipment used in the patient care.

5. Determine the initial UVB dose (mJ/cm^2) according to the patient's skin type as classified by the physician. See Appendix for definitions of skin types.

Skin Type	Initial UVB Dose (mJ/cm^2)
Type I	20
Type II	25
Type III	30
Type IV	40
Type V	50
Type VI	60

6. The manual method for calculation of the time (seconds) to set the UVB control panel to deliver the dose from #5 is the following equation: (The measurement of the irradiance can be obtained from the logbook kept on a weekly basis.)

$$\text{Time (seconds)} = \text{Dose (mJ/cm}^2) \div \text{Irradiance (mW/cm}^2)$$

7. The duration of a treatment or total dose of UVB to be delivered can often be calculated by the UV light unit by following the manufacturer's instructions in the operations manual and inputting the correct information on the control panel prior to the delivery of the treatment.

8. Set the time (or dose) on the control panel of the UV light unit and on the additional safety timer kept in the light unit or by the technician. In some phototherapy units, the session duration is dependent on the dose measured by an internal photometer, and the time must be estimated by the technician.

9. Verify that the UV light unit is set on UVB.

10. Turn on the fan and have the patient stand in the center of the UV light unit with their arms at rest. Double-check that they are wearing UV goggles as eye protection.

11. Instruct the patient to come out of the UV light box when the lights go out or if they become uncomfortable during the treatment either from burning or stinging of the skin. Inform the patient that the light-box doors are not locked.

12. Start the treatment.

13. Some patients may receive localized UV light therapy to the legs or trunk as ordered by the physician.

14. After completion of the UVB light treatment, the patient will be brought to the treatment area of the PTC. The nursing staff will apply anthralin paste to the areas of psoriasis avoiding the face, body folds, groin, and genitalia. All patients will start with 0.1% anthralin paste. First, the normal skin surrounding the plaques will be coated with Vaseline petroleum jelly for protection. Then, the anthralin paste will be applied. Talcum powder will be patted on the lesions to help prevent spread of the anthralin. Then, the areas are wrapped with saran wrap and a layer of cotton gauze over the saran wrap.

15. When application of the anthralin is completed, the patient is to be wrapped with saran wrap and this is to be secured in place. The patient is then to put on a surgical scrub suit supplied by the PTC. An alternative to wrapping with saran wrap followed by a surgical scrub suit is to use an occlusive garment that has proper fitting at the neck, wrists, and ankles. The areas treated with anthralin should still be wrapped with cotton gauze. A nylon or plastic body suit designed for this purpose can be acquired commercially.

16. There is to be at least 1–2 hours of anthralin under occlusion each day of Ingram treatment. The usual time required is 2 hours of occlusion unless otherwise specified by the attending physician.

17. The PTC lounge is provided for patients during this time of occlusion.

18. Scalp debridement therapy may be performed during the 2 hour period that patients are at the treatment center. See the protocol for scalp debridement.

19. At the end of the contact time with anthralin, the patient will use the shower or have a hydrosound bath (if ordered) to wash off the anthralin.

20. Ingram treatment patients are asked to apply a heavy emollient or Aquaphor ointment to the involved areas at night and leave on overnight.

SUBSEQUENT TREATMENTS

21. The frequency of Ingram treatments for the diagnosis of psoriasis is 5 times a week unless otherwise ordered by a physician. If less than 4 times a week has been ordered, then special instructions for the advancement of the dose of UVB light must accompany the request.

22. On subsequent visits, the patient will be asked about redness, light pink color, and tenderness of the skin the previous night, and this information will be put into the phototherapy record.

23. If the skin is red, the phototherapist will ask that the patient be seen by the attending physician who will make the decision for adjustment in the treatment for that day. If the skin is a light pink color, the phototherapist should keep the dose the same as the previously delivered treatment dose.

24. Increase the dose (mJ/cm^2) of the UVB light by the amount as follows, and add it to the previous dose delivered to the patient if the treatment has been within 3 days:

Skin Type	Amount of UVB Increase (mJ/cm^2)
Type I	5
Type II	10
Type III	15
Type IV	20
Type V	25
Type VI	30

25. For subsequent treatments, these corresponding steps can be done if the following time between treatments have been observed:

4–7 days	Keep the dose the same.
1–2 weeks	Decrease the dose by 25%.
2–3 weeks	Decrease the dose by 50%.
3–4 weeks	Decrease the dose by 75%.
More than 4 weeks	Start over

26. Increase the strength of anthralin according to the following table as treatment progresses. If irritation, accompanied by tenderness or pain, develops at the site of the anthralin applications, then the physician will need to be notified and the strength adjusted.

Days of Treatment	Strength of Anthralin (%)
1–3	0.1
4–6	0.25
7–9	0.5
10–12	1.0
13–15	2.0
16–18	3.0
19–21	4.0

27. Follow steps 6–20 previously.

LOCALIZED DELIVERY OF ULTRAVIOLET B

PATIENT INSTRUCTIONS FOR EXCIMER LASER AT 308 NM WAVELENGTH

1. Localized, or recalcitrant plaque-type psoriasis may be treated with the excimer laser through delivery of 308 nm UV light from the excimer laser. This type of phototherapy may be used alone, or in combination with other treatments.

2. All patients designated to receive excimer laser therapy will have the routine introduction to the PTC facility.

3. All patients designated to receive excimer laser therapy will have the basic introduction to the laser equipment and safety procedures. Appropriate contact information for the PTC is to be given to the patient.

4. Initial therapy with the excimer laser is twice weekly. The frequency of treatments may decrease if the response to treatment is adequate.

5. Instruct patient to wear protective eye glasses while undergoing treatments.

6. Instruct patients that the procedure is typically pain-free and to remain still while the treatment is administered. Warn them that they may feel a sensation of warmth.

7. The patient's current medication list will be placed in the patient's chart and reviewed by the phototherapist. Medication-related questions will be addressed by the attending physician.

8. All patients will be told of the possible complications of excimer laser therapy:

    a.   Sunburn reaction
    b.   Eye damage (corneal burns)
    c.   Freckling
    d.   Pigmentation changes
    e.   Possible increased risk of skin cancers
    f.   Possible premature aging effects

9. Patients will be given UVB phototherapy brochures and brochures from the National Psoriasis Foundation if they have not previously received them.

PROTOCOL

1. Obtain a signed consent form after the patient has been given the tour of the PTC and the appropriate education and safety instructions.

2. Prior to the initiation of excimer laser treatments, the patient will be asked to attend the treatment center for determination of the MED. The agenda for the first patient visit is as follows:

    a. Obtain a patient history
    b. Pretreatment photographs, if desired
    c. Determination of Fitzpatrick skin type
    d. MED test

3. Determine the MED using the following procedure*:

    a. Place the appropriate template that accompanies the laser device on an area of sun-protected skin, typically the hip or buttocks.
    b. Mark the orientation of the template to ensure accurate interpretation of the MED.
    c. The patient is to wear protective glasses/goggles during delivery of the UV doses for the MED testing.
    d. Refer to the appropriate protocol accompanying your laser device for MED testing. Typical doses for MED testing are 100, 150, 200, 250, 300, and 350 mJ/cm^2 and correspond to dosing levels of 1–6, respectively.

Dosing Value	Dose (mJ/cm^2)
1	100
2	150
3	200
4	250
5	300
6	350

    e. The patient is to return for determination of their MED 24 hours after delivery of the UV light.
    f. The dose that corresponds to the first area with detectable erythema or pinkness from the MED test is defined as the MED.
    g. The MED is to be recorded in the phototherapy treatment record.

---

* Adapted from XTRAC XL Plus Excimer Laser Phototherapy System, In-service training manual, Photomedex, Carlsbad, CA.

Fitzpatrick Skin Types

Skin Type	Sunburn/Tanning History
I	Always burns, never tans; sensitive ("Celtic")
II	Burns easily, tans rarely
III	Burns moderately, tans gradually to light brown
IV	Burns minimally, always tans well to moderately brown (olive skin)
V	Rarely burns, tans profusely to dark brown (brown skin)
VI	Never burns, deeply pigmented; not sensitive (black skin)

Source: Fitzpatrick, T.B., *Arch. Dermatol.*, 124, 869, 1988.

4. Patient's skin must be free of lotions, makeup, deodorant, etc.

5. Wipe plaques lightly with mineral oil.

6. Treatment dosing is based on multiples of the MED (i.e., the MED multiplier). For example, a 3 MED dose equals a dose of light 3 times the determined MED dose; for a patient with an MED of 3 (200 mJ/cm^2), a 3 MED dose is 3 times 200 or 600 mJ/cm^2.*

7. The MED multiplier is based on plaque characteristics and location. Knees, elbows, hands, and feet are initially treated with 3 MED, or 3 times the MED. All other areas are initially treated with 2 MED, or 2 times the MED. For thick plaques, the MED multiplier may be increased by 1. For thin plaques, the MED multiplier may be reduced by 1. For tan plaques, the MED multiplier may be increased by 1. Refer to the manufacturer's operation manual for further, specific operating instructions.

8. Special care should be given to the wrists, dorsum of hands, ankles, and feet as these areas may burn easily.

9. The frequency of treatments is twice a week.

10. Subsequent (follow-up) dosing is determined by response to the most recent treatment:

    a. If there is/was considerable burning or any blistering, reduce MED multiplier by 1 and avoid treatment of injured area.
    b. If there is not considerable improvement of the treated area, and no burning/blistering is seen, increase MED multiplier by 1.

11. Always instruct patients to avoid natural UV light exposure to treated areas and to apply antibiotic ointment should blistering occur and to not disrupt the blister itself.

12. Ensure that the patient has the contact information of the PTC for any questions/concerns.

---

* A laser-specific protocol typically accompanies the device. Refer to specific manufacturer's instructions for operation and safety features of the device.

PATIENT INSTRUCTIONS FOR HANDHELD UVB DEVICES

1. Localized, or recalcitrant plaque-type psoriasis may be treated using a limited spectrum of UVB delivered from a filamentous light source through a handheld delivery system. Localized phototherapy may be used alone or in combination with other treatments.

2. All patients designated to receive localized UVB phototherapy will have the routine introduction to the PTC facility.

3. All patients designated to receive localized UVB phototherapy will have the basic introduction to the equipment and safety procedures. Appropriate contact information for the PTC is to be given to the patient.

4. Initially, localized UVB phototherapy sessions will be performed 2–3 times weekly on nonconsecutive days. Patients having fewer than two treatments a week will need to have instructions from a physician.

5. Instruct patient to wear protective eyeglasses while undergoing treatments.

6. Instruct patients that the procedure is typically pain-free and to remain still while the treatment is administered. Warn them that they may feel a sensation of warmth.

7. The patient's current medication list will be placed in the patient's chart and reviewed by the phototherapist. Medication-related questions will be addressed by the attending physician.

8. All patients will be told of the possible complication of localized UVB therapy:

    a. Sunburn reaction
    b. Eye damage (corneal burns)
    c. Freckling
    d. Pigmentation changes
    e. Possible increased risk of skin cancers
    f. Possible premature aging effects

9. Patients will be given a UVB phototherapy brochure and brochures from the National Psoriasis Foundation if they have not previously received them.

PROTOCOL

1. Obtain a signed consent form after the patient has been given the tour of the PTC and the appropriate education and safety instruction.

2. Prior to the initiation of localized UVB treatments, the patient will be asked to attend the treatment center for determination of the MED. The agenda for the first patient visit is as follows:

    a. Obtain a patient history
    b. Pretreatment photographs, if desired
    c. Determination of Fitzpatrick skin type
    d. MED dose delivery

3. Determine the MED using the following procedure:
    a. The patient and operator are to wear protective glasses/goggles during delivery of the UV doses for the MED testing.
    b. Define the patient's Fitzpatrick skin type in accordance with the following table.

Fitzpatrick Skin Types

Skin Type	Sunburn/Tanning History
I	Always burns, never tans; sensitive ("Celtic")
II	Burns easily, tans rarely
III	Burns moderately, tans gradually to light brown
IV	Burns minimally, always tans well to moderately brown (olive skin)
V	Rarely burns, tans profusely to dark brown (brown skin)
VI	Never burns, deeply pigmented; not sensitive (black skin)

Source: Fitzpatrick, T.B., *Arch. Dermatol.*, 124, 869, 1988.

    c. Mark six skin patch locations (2 cm × 2 cm each) that will be used for MED testing in an appropriate area of sun-protected skin, such as the hip or buttocks.
    d. Refer to the operation manual from the manufacturer for the proper methods to select and deliver a UVB dose.
    e. The following six UVB doses will be delivered in accordance with the patient's skin type:

Ultraviolet B Phototest Doses (mJ/cm²) by Skin Type

Dose Sequence	Skin Type					
	I	II	III	IV	V	VI
First	40	70	90	120	150	180
Second	60	90	120	150	180	210
Third	70	105	150	180	210	240
Fourth	90	120	180	210	240	270
Fifth	105	150	210	240	270	300
Sixth	120	180	240	270	300	330

f. The patient is to return for determination of their MED 24 hours after delivery of the UVB.

g. The skin patch that corresponds to the lowest dose-producing erythema or pinkness is defined as the MED.

h. The MED is to be recorded in the phototherapy treatment record.

4. Patient's skin must be free of lotions, makeup, deodorant, etc.

5. Wipe plaques lightly with mineral oil.

6. Treatment dosing is based on multiples of the MED (i.e., the MED multiplier). The multiplier to be used during treatment is based upon plaque characteristics and location. In general, the objective will be to utilize as high a UVB dose as can be tolerated by the skin, while avoiding symptomatic sunburn-like reactions and blistering of the skin.

7. Treatment frequency is twice a week. Close monitoring for the changes that occur at the treatment sites is necessary to be able to determine whether an increase or decrease in the MED multiplier is indicated.

8. Typical UVB dose setting strategies are as follows:

Typical Targeted Ultraviolet B Dose Setting Strategies

| Location | Scale/Induration | Initial Dose (First 2–3 Treatments) | | Subsequent Dose |
		2 Treatments per Week	3 Treatments per Week	
Elbows/knees/fingers	Moderate	6 MEDs	5 MEDs	Adjust up/down[a]
	Slight	4 MEDs	4 MEDs	Adjust up/down[a]
Back/trunk/limbs	Moderate	4 MEDs	3 MEDs	Adjust up/down[a]
	Slight	3 MEDs	2 MEDs	Adjust up/down[a]
Scalp	Moderate	4 MEDs	3 MEDs	Adjust up/down[a]
	Slight	3 MEDs	2 MEDs	Adjust up/down[a]

[a] Utilize as high a UVB dose as can be tolerated by the skin, while avoiding symptomatic erythema and blister formation.

9. Special care should be given to the wrists, dorsum of hands, ankles, and dorsum of feet as these areas may burn easily.

10. Always instruct patients to avoid natural UV light exposure to treated areas and to apply antibiotic ointment should blistering occur and to avoid disrupting the blister itself.

11. Ensure that the patient has the contact information of the PTC for any questions/concerns.

HOME NARROWBAND ULTRAVIOLET B PHOTOTHERAPY

The use of therapeutic phototherapy in the home location is an important consideration for the proper patient. This section will be focused on use of home NBUVB units serving as home delivery devices for treatment of psoriasis compared to office or an outpatient treatment facility. The discussion and protocols related to home UV therapy are for medical devices and not for commercial tanning bed equipment. While some lamps used in the tanning salon industry do contain small amounts of UVB wavelengths in their spectrum, if a physician is to prescribe home UV delivery systems it should be for the medical treatment of a disease process with the proper equipment, medical UV source, known effectiveness, and with appropriate safety precautions.

CANDIDATES FOR HOME PHOTOTHERAPY

Psoriasis is the primary disease consideration for NBUVB therapy whether in the clinic setting or at home. This manual considers many other diseases for application of phototherapy protocols with the understanding the treatments would be done in a setting of continued assessment and delivery by trained professionals. The chronic nature of psoriasis and need for ongoing therapy over time in consideration with the proven effectiveness of NBUVB as a treatment makes psoriasis the primary disease process selected for home UV therapy. Vitiligo is also a photoresponsive skin disease treated with NBUVB with proven benefit in some patients. However, the variability of response in different regions of the body, plus the greater likelihood of phototoxic reactions in the affected skin even in a controlled environment limits the application for home treatment except in selected cases with individualized protocols by the physician. The protocols for home NBUVB will be limited to psoriasis. I do not prescribe home NBUVB units to treat atopic dermatitis patients or for cutaneous lymphoma patients.

SELECTION OF PATIENTS

The best candidates for treatment of psoriasis in the home phototherapy setting are selected with one or more of the following parameters:

- Psoriasis with mild to moderate severity
- No photosensitive disorders
- No photosensitizing mediations
- Previous demonstrated effectiveness of UV light
  - Seasonal improvement from natural sunlight
  - Demonstrated response to office NBUVB treatment

- Limited or no access to clinic or facility due to
  - Travel distance
  - Work schedule
  - Time commitment
- Patient preference to avoid systemic medications either ingested or injected

EQUIPMENT

The protocols listed are for use with NBUVB units with six foot fluorescent lamps. There are many manufacturers in the United States and worldwide who produce high-quality equipment. The features of home phototherapy devices and the safety parameters engineered into their production have been a very positive aspect regarding the confidence with which a clinician can prescribe home phototherapy for their patients. Features include

- Household electrical supply adequate
- Same TL-01 lamps for NBUVB as used in office or clinic setting
- Efficient space saving panels with ease of mobility
- Digital input and codes to turn on device
- Programmed limited number of treatments with renewal through prescribing physician's office
- Emergency cut off switches
- Photometers as part of the package or built into the device

The use of other light sources in addition to production of NBUVB through six foot long fluorescent tubes have demonstrated efficacy for treatment of psoriasis, such as light-emitting diodes (LED). Specifically, there are some LED devices with blue light wavelengths used for treatment with innovative delivery systems for localized treatment and or sheets of LED light to lay over the skin or region of the body. This discussion is limited to the NBUVB home phototherapy treatment devices. Further discussion on the use of and treatment with handheld and localized delivery of phototherapy is contained in separate chapters of this manual.

PATIENT INSTRUCTIONS

1. Recalcitrant plaque-type psoriasis may be treated with UV light from a narrowband UVB (NBUVB) unit placed in the home. This type of phototherapy may be used alone, or in combination with other treatments.

2. All patients designated for home NBUVB phototherapy will receive the appropriate contact information for the PTC.

3. Initial therapy with the home NBUVB unit may vary from 3 to 4 times per week. The frequency of treatments is dependent upon the resistance of the case of psoriasis and the physician's recommendations.

4. You must take the necessary protective measures while undergoing treatments, including wearing protective eyewear, properly covering of the areas such as the genitals, and when applicable, the face.

5. The procedure is typically pain-free and you should remain still while the treatment is administered. It is OK to move your arms while being treated, but you should stand in one place during the treatment. You may feel a sensation of warmth during the treatment.

6. A current medication list will be placed in the patient's chart and reviewed by the phototherapist. Medication-related questions will be addressed by the attending physician.

7. All patients will be told of the possible complication of home NBUVB phototherapy including

    a. Sunburn reaction
    b. Eye damage (corneal burns)
    c. Photoallergic dermatitis (including drug reactions)
    d. Freckling
    e. Pigmentation changes
    f. Possible increased risk of skin cancers
    g. Aging effects of UVB light

8. Patients will be given UVB phototherapy brochures and brochures from the National Psoriasis Foundation if they have not previously received them.

9. The manufacturer's instructions for the setup and operation of the NBUVB home unit must be followed.

PROTOCOL

1. Before starting therapy, you must consult a physician regarding your skin type and to obtain an individualized treatment plan including a starting dose.

2. The goal of NBUVB phototherapy treatment is to achieve 75% clearing within a period of several weeks without experiencing reddening or burning of the skin. A painless "pinkening" of the skin is acceptable. NBUVB works by delivering light to the skin. Light is a form of energy. The time of exposure to the light determines the total amount of energy delivered.

3. Skin that is to be treated must be free of lotions, makeup, deodorant, etc.

4. Apply a thin layer of mineral oil to the areas of psoriasis.

5. Males must wear covering over the genitals while undergoing treatment.

6. Eye protection in the form of UV goggles must be worn at all times when the phototherapy unit is activated.

7. The amount of light is highly dependent on how close you stand to the unit. Stand 1 foot away from the unit. You much be consistent. It may help to place a mark or piece of masking tape on the floor to ensure you are in the same spot each time.

8. Initial exposure times are based on a determination of an amount of UV light. Consider it a dose of medication. In this case, the medicine is the UV light. The dose is dependent upon your skin type and MED as indicated by the prescribing physician. The following table may be used as a reference:

Fitzpatrick Skin Type

Skin Type	Sunburn/Tanning History
I	Always burns, never tans; sensitive ("Celtic")
II	Burns easily, tans rarely
III	Burns moderately, tans gradually to light brown
IV	Burns minimally, always tans well to moderately brown (olive skin)
V	Rarely burns, tans profusely to dark brown (brown skin)
VI	Never burns, deeply pigmented; not sensitive (black skin)

Source: Fitzpatrick, T.B., Arch. Dermatol., 124, 869, 1988.

Listed in the following table are generally accepted starting doses of NBUVB light based on skin type. It is very important to understand that these doses are only to be used for the special NBUVB light. If you have questions about what light you have for your home use, ask your physician.

Skin Type	Initial Dose (mJ/cm²)
Type I	120
Type II	140
Type III	160
Type IV	180
Type V	200
Type VI	220

The amount of time necessary to give a specific dose of NBUVB light will depend on your specific NBUVB home light box and what the manufacturer's specifications are for that unit. Most new units produced today use the dose as the determining factor and the machine calculates how long that will take. Refer to the manufacturer's operation manual or the dosing chart that comes with the NBUVB unit to find the amount of time necessary for the dose to be given.

9. Subsequent (follow-up) dosing is determined by the response to the most recent treatment. If pinkening of skin (slight erythema) occurs from the last treatment, maintain last treatment time. If reddening or sunburn occurs, stop treatment until the reddening dissipates, and then start at one-half of the previous dose.

10. Subsequent increases after the first treatment should be made in small increments. Any increase should be based on reaction to the previous treatment. Increases in the dose should be made only if NO erythema or pinkening occurred from the most recent dose. Recommended increases in the NBUVB dose can be found in the following table:

Skin Type	Increase in NBUVB Dose (mJ/cm²)
Type I	10
Type II	20
Type III	20
Type IV	30
Type V	30
Type VI	40

11. The frequency of initial treatments should be either 3 times a week (M, W, F) or 4 times a week (M, T, Th, F) as determined by your prescribing physician. A chart with the date of treatment and the dose last given should be kept for every treatment session.

12. Once you have acceptable improvement in your degree of psoriasis, typically in about 20–30 treatments, a maintenance regimen can be started. Maintenance therapy typically involves one to two treatments per week. If clearing continues, one treatment every 7–10 days may suffice. You may discontinue treatment if your skin clears and remains clear for 1–3 months during the maintenance therapy.

13. If your psoriasis becomes active, revert back to the previous treatment schedule. For example, once-a-week maintenance treatments would increase in frequency to treatments of twice a week for 2–3 weeks as may be determined by your physician.

14. If your psoriasis becomes active and you have been off NBUVB phototherapy for months, you will have to start over at the beginning of the treatment schedule and build up the dose again.

15. Not all home NBUVB phototherapy units have the same number of bulbs or need the same amount of time to produce the dose that you may need to start and continue therapy. It is very important to follow the manufacturer's operational manual and to ask questions of the manufacturer and/or your physician if you are uncertain of the treatments.

SPECIALIZED TREATMENTS

PROTOCOL FOR HAND AND/OR FOOT TREATMENTS

1. Hand and foot treatments may be given in specialized hand and foot units, or with the standard UVA/UVB phototherapy units. They may be given alone or in combination with total body treatments.

2. If hand and foot treatments are given in combination with total body treatments, patients may dress after their body treatment and before their hand and foot treatments.

3. Instruct patient to wear protective glasses for eye protection while undergoing treatments.

4. If using standard UVA/UVB phototherapy units, care should be taken to cover/drape all untreated areas.

5. Special care should be given to the wrists, dorsum of hands, ankles, and dorsum of feet. These areas burn easily and may require sunscreen or covering with layers of cloth for protection.

6. For UVA dosing, follow the same protocol for UVA phototherapy for the specific disease being treated.

7. For UVB dosing, follow the same protocol for UVB phototherapy for the specific disease being treated.

8. For NBUVB dosing to the palms and soles, assume a MED of 1000 mJ/cm^2, and then follow the same protocol for UVB phototherapy for the specific disease being treated.

PATIENT INSTRUCTIONS FOR SCALP DEBRIDEMENT

1. All patients designated for the scalp debridement protocol will be given the routine introduction to the PTC.

2. All patients designated for the scalp debridement protocol will have the basic introduction to the scalp debridement unit (SDU) and shown its operation.

3. Patients selected for treatment must be able to lie flat and extend their head without discomfort.

4. To prepare for the treatments, the patients should wear a gown over their clothes or have a covering to protect their clothing during the treatment period.

5. A shower cap will be provided to the patient during the 30-minute time period after the application of anthralin and removal of the medication.

6. All patients will be told of the possible complications of anthralin therapy including

    a. Irritation of the skin at the site of application.
    b. Staining of the skin (a purple color) at the site of the location.
    c. Staining of the hair (a purple color), which comes into contact with the anthralin. This is especially problematic for patients with light hair color.
    d. Staining of clothing, which has contact with the anthralin medication.

7. The frequency of the treatment will be determined by the physician with routine initiation of treatment being 2 times a week.

PROTOCOL

1. The patient will have time for questions after the orientation to the PTC and the SDU or the scalp treatment area with treatment basin.

2. Prior to the initial segment of the treatment, the patient will remove their outer shirt and leave undergarments in place. A scrub shirt or smock will be provided to them to use during the course of the treatment.

3. Either an SDU or a specialized sink with a flexible handheld nozzle for rinsing the scalp should be available.

4. The patient will lie with the neck extended and place the head into a basin or into the SDU for the initial rinse.

5. A rinse cycle should be carried out prior to application of any medications to moisten the scalp and loosen the adherent scale.

6. Direct application of a salicylic acid preparation or a phenol and salicylic acid preparation can be used to aid in the debridement process.

7. An additional rinse may be required to remove any residual material from the scalp.

8. Manual application of Micanol® or 1% anthralin cream to the involved areas of psoriasis is to be done by the technician. Care should be taken not to let this spread to the neck or on the face during the process.

9. A plastic shower cap is to be applied over the scalp with gauze covering the areas of skin that may be involved with psoriasis at the hairline and touching occluded by the shower cap.

10. The patient should then wait 30 minutes after application of the anthralin. A handheld timer should be used to set the time and the patient should also be told the time when the next segment of treatment is expected to start.

11. At the end of the 30-minute anthralin contact time, the patient will again be placed into the SDU for a full cycle of rinse, shampoo, rinse to aid in the removal of the anthralin.

12. Following the partial removal of the anthralin with the SDU, the technician will use manual application of triethanolamine to all areas where anthralin was used. This is applied in the form of a spray and massaged into the areas.

13. An additional rinse will need to be done after the use of triethanolamine.

14. Other hair products such as creme rinses or hair conditioners may be used after the final rinse cycle.

15. During the days that the patient has not received a scalp treatment for psoriasis, routine use of a psoriasis shampoo and topical corticosteroid solutions after rinsing is to be made part of their home therapy.

PATIENT INSTRUCTIONS FOR HYDROSOUND BATH

1. Show patient the hydrosound bath room.

2. Explain to the patient how to use the emergency call light.

3. The patient will be told they may undress in the bath area or use the locker area and wear a robe into the hydrosound bath area.

4. Patients must be told they are to be in the tub for 15 minutes unless they have uncomfortable ringing in their ears or stinging of their skin.

5. Instruct male patients to wear swim trunks or an athletic supporter.

6. Patients will be asked to enter the tub with assistance. If there is any difficulty stepping into the tub the patient lift is available for their use.

PROTOCOL

1. Fill tank with water (95°F) above the ultrasound plate. Place rubber mat in the bottom of the tub.

2. Add hydrosound water conditioner to the tub water by pumping the measured dispenser three times into the tub.

3. Turn timer to 20 minutes with intensity of 100, to de-gas the water as per the instructions from the manufacturer.

4. Assist patient into the tub, using the patient lift if the patient has any difficulty stepping into the tub. Patients must be able to stand unassisted to be able to use the patient lift and to be considered for hydrosound therapy.

5. Turn hydrosound timer on. The standard length of time for a hydrosound bath is 15 minutes. The time may be adjusted as per the physician's orders.

6. Set the timer on the hydrosound control panel to 15 minutes.

7. Leave the intensity at 100 unless the patient complains of ringing in the ears or stinging on the skin. The intensity may then be adjusted to 80. If the ringing in the ears or stinging is still uncomfortable to the patient then the treatment is to be stopped and the physician notified.

8. The patients will be attended by PTC personnel either in the room or in the hallway of the bath facility with the door open throughout the duration of the hydrosound bath.

9. Assist patient out of the tub at the end of the treatment.

10. Drain the water from the tub.

11. Clean the tub per manufacturer's instructions with disinfectant solution, using a cloth to wipe down the tub. Let stand a few minutes, and then rinse.

REFERENCE
Fitzpatrick TB. The validity and practicality of sun-reactive types I through VI. *Arch. Dermatol.*, 124, 869–871, 1988.

Vitiligo

NARROWBAND ULTRAVIOLET B PHOTOTHERAPY

PATIENT INSTRUCTIONS

1. All patients designated for the narrowband ultraviolet B (NBUVB) protocol for treatment of vitiligo will have the routine introduction to the Phototherapy Treatment Center (PTC) facility.

2. All patients designated for the NBUVB protocol for the treatment of vitiligo will have the basic introduction to phototherapy equipment and safety procedures.

3. Reinforcement of the need for eye protection for all patients and covering of the genital area in males is required.

4. Patients are to stand in the center of the light cabinet with their arms at rest. A step stool may be used for the patients to stand on when recommended by the physician.

5. A handheld timer will be set by the phototherapy technician for each treatment session. The time will correspond to the estimated time of the treatment session duration, and the timer will either be given to the patient to have with them during the treatment session or be kept by the technician during the treatment. The time will correspond with the amount of time calculated for their dose of NBUVB for that treatment.

6. Instruct patients to come out of the light box when the lights have gone out or within 10 seconds of the alarm of the safety (handheld) timer. Inform patients that the light-box doors are not locked and demonstrate their operation.

7. The list of current medications will be placed in the patient's chart and reviewed by the phototherapist. Questions concerning current medications will be addressed by the attending physician.

8. All patients will be told of the possible complications of NBUVB phototherapy specifically including

    a. Sunburn reaction
    b. Corneal burn if the eyes are unprotected
    c. Photoallergic dermatitis (including drug reaction)
    d. Freckling of the skin
    e. Aging of the skin
    f. Possible increase in risk of skin cancers

9. Patients will be told that additional unprotected sun exposure should be avoided on the days they receive NBUVB. Sunblock (SPF 15) should be used on any sun-exposed areas for the remainder of that day.

10. All patients will be given the brochure on UVB phototherapy from the National Psoriasis Foundation.

PROTOCOL

1.   Obtain a signed consent form after the patient has been given the tour of the PTC and basic phototherapy education concerning NBUVB phototherapy. The patient should be given time for questions.

2.   Have the patient undress and expose the areas of vitiligo to be treated. Clothing or cloth covering may be used to shield the normal skin. Male patients should wear an athletic supporter unless otherwise directed or permitted by the attending physician.

3.   Eye protection in the form of ultraviolet (UV) goggles must be worn by all patients when inside the phototherapy unit.

4.   The irradiance (mW/cm^2) of the NBUVB light inside the unit should be recorded on a once-a-month basis using the standard method of the manufacturer of the phototherapy unit. Record this irradiance on the phototherapy record sheet or keep an irradiance logbook for the equipment used in patient care.

5.   The initial NBUVB dose (mJ/cm^2) will be the same for all patients with vitiligo. It is 300 mJ/cm^2.

6.   The manual method for calculation of the time (seconds) to set the NBUVB control panel to deliver the dose from #5 is the following equation: (The measurement of the irradiance can be obtained from the logbook kept on a weekly basis.)

$$\text{Time (seconds)} = \text{Dose (mJ/cm}^2) \div \text{Irradiance (mW/cm}^2)$$

7.   The duration of a treatment or total dose of NBUVB to be delivered can often be calculated by the UV light unit by following the manufacturer's instructions in the operations manual and inputting the correct information on the control panel prior to the delivery of the treatment.

8.   Set the time (or dose) on the control panel of the UV light unit and on the additional safety timer kept in the light unit or by the technician. In some phototherapy units, the session duration is dependent on the dose measured by an internal photometer and the time must be estimated by the technician.

9.   Verify that the UV light unit is set on NBUVB.

10. Turn on the fan and have the patient stand in the center of the UV light unit with their arms at rest. Double-check that they are wearing UV goggles as eye protection.

11. Instruct the patient to come out of the UV light box when the lights go out or if they become uncomfortable during the treatment either from burning or stinging of the skin. Inform the patient that the light-box doors are not locked.

12. Start the treatment.

SUBSEQUENT TREATMENTS

13. The frequency of NBUVB light treatments for the diagnosis of vitiligo is 2 times a week unless otherwise ordered by a physician. If more than 2 times a week has been ordered by a physician, then special instructions for the advancement of the dose of NBUVB light must accompany the request.

14. On subsequent visits, the patient will be asked about redness, light pink color, and tenderness of the skin the previous night and this information will be put into the phototherapy record.

15. If the skin is red, the phototherapy technician will ask that the patient be seen by the attending physician who will make the decision for adjustment in the NBUVB treatment for that day. If the skin is a light pink color, the phototherapist should keep the dose the same as the previously delivered treatment dose.

16. Increase the UVB dose by the following amount until the patient reports that slight erythema is observed within 24 hours after treatment.

    Subsequent treatments—increase dose by 50 mJ/cm^2

17. Do not continue to increase the dose if slight erythema occurs within 24 hours after the last treatment. The erythema should not persist for 24 hours and should not sting or burn. If there is persistence of erythema or burning for 24 hours or longer, reduce the dose by 25%.

18. Do not exceed 600 mJ/cm^2 unless otherwise ordered by the physician.

19. For subsequent treatments, if the following time between treatments have been observed, these are the corresponding steps to be done:

4–7 days	Keep the dose the same.
1–2 weeks	Decrease the dose by 25%.
2–3 weeks	Decrease the dose by 50%.
More than 3 weeks	Start over.

20. Follow steps 6–12 previously.

LOCALIZED DELIVERY OF ULTRAVIOLET (UVB) EXCIMER LASER AT 308 NM WAVELENGTH

PATIENT INSTRUCTIONS

1. All patients designated to receive excimer laser phototherapy for the treatment of vitiligo will have the routine introduction to the PTC facility.

2. All patients designated to receive excimer laser phototherapy will have the basic introduction to the equipment and safety procedures. Appropriate contact information for the PTC is to be given to the patient.

3. Initially, excimer laser sessions will be performed twice weekly on non-consecutive days. The frequency of treatments may increase or decrease, depending upon the rate of repigmentation.

4. Instruct patient to wear protective eye glasses while undergoing treatments.

5. Instruct patients that the procedure is typically pain-free and to remain still while the treatment is administered. Warn them that they may feel a sensation of warmth.

6. The patient's current medication list with be placed in the patient's chart and reviewed by the phototherapist. Medication-related questions will be addressed by the attending physician.

7. All patients will be told of the possible complication of excimer laser treatments including

   a. Sunburn reaction
   b. Eye damage (corneal burns)
   c. Freckling
   d. Pigmentation changes
   e. Possible increased risk of skin cancers
   f. Possible premature aging effects

8. Patients will be given UVB phototherapy brochures and brochures concerning information on vitiligo if they have not previously received them.

PROTOCOL

1. Obtain a signed consent form after the patient has been given the tour of the PTC and the appropriate education and safety instructions.

2. Patient's skin must be free of lotions, makeup, deodorant, etc.

3. Initiate treatment using an excimer laser dose of 200 mJ/cm^2. Refer to the operation manual of the device supplied by the manufacturer to select the dose and for the proper delivery of the laser light.

4. For subsequent treatments, increase the UVB dose by 50 mJ/cm^2 until the patient reports that slight erythema is observed within 24 hours after treatment.

5. Maintain dosage used to produce slight erythema. The erythema should not persist for 24 hours and should not sting or burn. If there is persistence of erythema or burning for 24 hours or longer, reduce the dose by 25%.

6. If slight erythema stops occurring and there is no repigmentation, increase the dose by 20 mJ/cm^2 and question the patient about the production of slight erythema within 24 hours after treatment. Continue to increase dosage by 20 mJ/cm^2 until a slight erythema is produced within 24 hours after treatment.

7. Do not exceed 800 mJ/cm^2 unless ordered by the attending physician.

8. Instruct patients to avoid natural UV light exposure to treated areas and to apply antibiotic ointment should blistering occur and to avoid disrupting the blister itself.

9. Ensure that the patient has the contact information of the PTC for any questions/concerns.

HANDHELD DEVICES

PATIENT INSTRUCTIONS

1. All patients designated to receive localized UVB phototherapy will have the routine introduction to the PTC facility.

2. All patients designated to receive localized UVB phototherapy will have the basic introduction to the equipment and safety procedures. Appropriate contact information for the PTC is to be given to the patient.

3. Initially, localized UVB phototherapy sessions will be performed twice weekly on nonconsecutive days. The frequency of treatments may increase or decrease, depending upon the rate of repigmentation.

4. Instruct patient to wear protective eye glasses while undergoing treatments.

5. Instruct patients that the procedure is typically pain-free and to remain still while the treatment is administered. Warn them that they may feel a sensation of warmth.

6. The patient's current medication list will be placed in the patient's chart and reviewed by the phototherapist. Medication-related questions will be addressed by the attending physician.

7. All patients will be told of the possible complication of localized UVB therapy:

   a. Sunburn reaction
   b. Eye damage (corneal burns)
   c. Freckling
   d. Pigmentation changes
   e. Possible increased risk of skin cancers
   f. Possible premature aging effects

8. Patients will be given UVB phototherapy brochures and brochures concerning information on vitiligo if they have not previously received them.

PROTOCOL

1. Obtain a signed consent form after the patient has been given the tour of the PTC and the appropriate education and safety instruction.

2. Patient's skin must be free of lotions, makeup, deodorant, etc.

3. Initiate treatment using a UVB dose of 90 mJ/cm^2. Refer to the operation manual of the device supplied by the manufacturer to select the dose and for the proper delivery of the UVB light.

4. For subsequent treatments, increase the UVB dose by 20 mJ/cm^2 until the patient reports that slight erythema is observed within 24 hours after treatment.

5. Maintain the dosage used to produce a slight erythema. The erythema should not persist for 24 hours and should not sting or burn. If there is persistence of erythema or burning for 24 hours or longer, reduce the dose by 25%.

6. If slight erythema does not occur at all, increase the dose by 2C mJ/cm^2 and question the patient about the production of slight erythema within 24 hours after treatment. Continue to increase dosage by 20 mJ/cm^2 until a slight erythema is produced within 24 hours after treatment.

7. Instruct patients to avoid natural UV light exposure to treated areas, to apply antibiotic ointment should blistering occur, and to avoid disrupting the blister itself.

8. Ensure that the patient has the contact information of the PTC for any questions/concerns.

SYSTEMIC PSORALEN PLUS ULTRAVIOLET A TREATMENT

1. All patients designated for psoralen plus ultraviolet A (PUVA) will have the routine introduction to the PTC facility.

2. All patients designated for PUVA will have the basic introduction to phototherapy equipment and safety procedures.

3. Reinforcement of the need for eye protection for all patients and covering of the genital area in males is required.

4. Patients receiving systemic PUVA will be instructed to take Oxsoralen Ultra® tablets in the dose prescribed by their physician 1 hour prior to the estimated time of their arrival at the PTC. The treatment will be given between 1 hour 15 minutes and 1 hour 45 minutes after ingestion of the medication.

5. All patients ingesting Oxsoralen Ultra must wear protective UV-blocking glasses when outside, riding in a car, or next to a window from the time they take the medication and for the next 18–24 hours during daylight.

6. Patients are to stand in the center of the light cabinet with their arms at rest. A step stool may be used for the patient to stand on when recommended by the physician.

7. A handheld timer will be set by the phototherapy technician for each treatment session. The time will correspond to the estimated time of the treatment session duration, and the timer will either be given to the patients to have with them during the treatment session or be kept by the technician during the treatment. The time will correspond with the amount of time calculated for their dose of UVA for that treatment.

8. Instruct patients to come out of the light box when the lights have gone out or within 10 seconds of the alarm of the safety (handheld) timer. Inform patients that the light-box doors are not locked and demonstrate their operation.

9. The list of current medications will be placed in the patient's chart and reviewed by the phototherapist. Questions concerning the current medications will be addressed by the attending physician.

10. All patients will be told of the possible complications of PUVA photo-therapy specifically including

    a.   Sunburn reaction
    b.   Corneal burn if the eyes are unprotected
    c.   Cataract formation if the eyes are unprotected
    d.   Photoallergic dermatitis (including drug reaction)
    e.   Freckling of the skin
    f.   Aging of the skin
    g.   Increase in risk of skin cancers including melanoma

11. Patients will be told that additional unprotected sun exposure should be avoided on the days they receive PUVA. Wide-spectrum sunblock (UVA/B) should be used on any sun-exposed areas for the remainder of that day.

12. All patients will be given the brochure on PUVA phototherapy from the National Psoriasis Foundation.

PROTOCOL

1. The diagnosis of vitiligo must be documented and on the chart at the time of referral to the PTC.

2. Obtain a signed consent form after the patient has been given the tour of the PTC and basic phototherapy education concerning PUVA phototherapy. The patient should be given time for questions.

3. Oxsoralen Ultra (8-methoxypsoralen) is to be ingested by the patient at least 1 hour prior to arrival at PTC. Treatments may be given anytime between 1 hour 15 minutes and 1 hour 45 minutes after ingestion.

4. Dosage of the Oxsoralen Ultra tablets is dependent on the orders of the attending physician and will vary from patient to patient. The dosage for use in the treatment of vitiligo is 0.5 mg/kg. Adjustments may be made to the dose of the Oxsoralen by the attending physician.

5. Ask the patient the dose and at what time they ingested their medication.

6. Have the patient undress so that all areas of vitiligo that are to be treated are exposed to the UV light. Clothing or cloth covering may be used to shield the normal skin. Male patients should wear an athletic supporter unless otherwise directed or permitted by the attending physician.

7. Eye protection in the form of UV goggles must be worn by all patients when inside the phototherapy unit. The only exception to this rule will be by physician orders.

8. The irradiance (mW/cm^2) of the UVA light inside the unit should be recorded on a once-a-month basis using the standard method of the manufacturer of the phototherapy unit. Record this irradiance on the phototherapy record sheet or keep an irradiance logbook for the equipment used in patient care.

9. The initial dose of UVA light for all vitiligo patients will be 1.0 J/cm^2.

10. The manual method for calculation of the time (seconds) to set the UVA control panel to deliver the dose from #9 is the following equation: (The measurement of the irradiance can be obtained from the logbook kept on a weekly basis.)

$$\text{Time (seconds)} = \text{Dose (mJ/cm}^2) \div \text{Irradiance (mW/cm}^2)$$

11. The duration of a treatment or total dose of UVA to be delivered can often be calculated by the UV light unit by following the manufacturer's instructions in the operations manual and inputting the correct information on the control panel prior to the delivery of the treatment.

12. Set the time (or dose) on the control panel of the UV light unit and on the additional safety timer kept in the light unit or by the technician. In some phototherapy units, the session duration is dependent on the dose measured by an internal photometer, and the time must be estimated by the technician.

13.   Verify that the UV light unit is set on UVA.

14.   Turn on the fan and have the patient stand in the center of the UV light unit with their arms at rest. Double-check that they are wearing UV goggles as eye protection.

15.   Instruct the patient to come out of the UV light box when the lights go out or if they become uncomfortable during the treatment either from burning or stinging of the skin. Inform the patient that the light-box doors are not locked.

16.   Start the treatment.

17.   Some patients may receive localized UV light therapy to the legs or trunk as ordered by the physician.

SUBSEQUENT TREATMENTS

18.   The frequency of PUVA treatments for the diagnosis of vitiligo is once or twice a week unless otherwise ordered by a physician. If less than once a week has been ordered, then special instructions for the advancement of the dose of UVA light must accompany the request.

19.   On subsequent visits, the patient will be asked about redness, light pink color, and tenderness of the skin the previous night, and this information will be put into the phototherapy record. The patient will also be asked at what time they took the Oxsoralen Ultra tablets.

20.   If the skin is red, the phototherapist will ask that the patient be seen by the attending physician who will make the decision for adjustment in the treatment for that day. If the skin is a light pink color, the phototherapist should keep the dose the same as the previously delivered treatment dose.

21.   Increase the UVA dose by the following amount until the patient reports that slight erythema is observed at the sites of vitiligo within 24 hours after treatment:

Subsequent treatments—increase by 0.5 J/cm^2

22.   Do not continue to increase the dose if slight erythema at the sites of vitiligo occurs within 24 hours after the last treatment. The erythema should not persist for 24 hours and should not sting or burn. If there is persistence of erythema or burning for 24 hours or longer, reduce the dose by 25%.

23.   Do not exceed a dose of 5 J/cm^2 unless ordered by the attending physician.

24.   Follow steps 3–22 previously.

25.   An ophthalmology examination should be performed prior to and every 6 months during PUVA treatment.

26.   Laboratory monitoring may be done at baseline and every 6 months.

PSORALEN BATHS OR SOAKS PLUS ULTRAVIOLET A (BATH PUVA)

PATIENT INSTRUCTIONS

1. All patients designated for bath PUVA will have the routine introduction to the PTC facility.

2. All patients designated for bath PUVA will have the basic introduction to phototherapy equipment and safety procedures.

3. Reinforcement of the need for eye protection during treatment is required.

4. A list of current medications will be placed in the patient's chart and reviewed by the phototherapist. Questions concerning the current medications will be addressed by the attending physician.

5. All patients will have the procedure explained to them and will be told of the possible complications of PUVA phototherapy specifically including

    a. Sunburn reaction
    b. Corneal burn if the eyes are unprotected
    c. Cataract formation if the eyes are unprotected
    d. Photoallergic dermatitis (including drug reaction)
    e. Freckling of the skin
    f. Aging of the skin
    g. Increase in risk of skin cancers including melanoma

6. Patients will be told that additional sunbathing should be avoided on the days they receive PUVA. Sunblock (UVA/B) should be used on any treated sun-exposed areas for the remainder of that day.

7. All patients will be given the brochure on PUVA phototherapy from the National Psoriasis Foundation.

PROTOCOL

1. Obtain a signed consent form after the patient has been given the tour of the PTC and basic phototherapy education concerning PUVA phototherapy. The patient should be given time for questions.

2. Dilute 1 mL of 8-methoxypsoralen solution (1 mg/mL standard solution) in 2 L of warm water in a basin, or dilute 10 mL of 0.1 mg/mL Trioxsalen (trimethylpsoralen in 95% ethyl alcohol) in 2 L of warm water, which must be agitated during soaking.

3. Soak the patient's hands and/or feet or area of the body to be treated such as the forearm for 15 minutes. Set a handheld timer to be kept with the patient during the soaking procedure. Dry the skin by patting the surface with a dry towel. Wrap the wrist with multiple layers of cloth to provide protection from UVA light—*optional.*

4. The initial dose for bath PUVA for all skin types is 0.5 J/cm^2 of UVA.

5. The irradiance (mW/cm^2) of the UVA light unit should be recorded on a once-a-month basis using the standard method of the manufacturer of the phototherapy unit. Record this irradiance on the phototherapy record sheet or keep an irradiance logbook for the equipment used in patient care.

6. The manual method for calculation of the time (seconds) to set the UV control panel to deliver the dose from #4 is the following equation: (The measurement of the irradiance can be obtained from the logbook kept on a weekly basis.)

$$\text{Time (seconds)} = \text{Dose (mJ/cm}^2) \div \text{Irradiance (mW/cm}^2)$$

7. The duration of a treatment or total dose of UV to be delivered can often be calculated by the UV light unit by following the manufacturer's instructions in the operations manual and inputting the correct information on the control panel prior to the delivery of the treatment.

8. Set the time (or dose) on the control panel of the UV light unit and on the additional safety timer kept in the light unit or by the technician. In some phototherapy units, the session duration is dependent on the dose measured by an internal photometer, and the time must be estimated by the technician.

9. Verify that the UV light unit is set on UVA.

10. Have the patient put on protective glasses during the phototherapy treatment session and for 1 hour after treatment.

11. Start the treatment.

12. After the UVA treatment is given, the patient must thoroughly wash the treated areas to remove any medication residue on the surface of the skin. Sunblock (UVA/B) is provided for the patient to apply as a precautionary measure to avoid additional UV exposure that day.

13. Instruct the patient to avoid excessive sunlight for the remainder of the day. A burn may not show up until 48 hours after treatment. Treatments are not usually given on 2 consecutive days. This allows the nurse to observe accurately for erythema.

SUBSEQUENT TREATMENTS

14. Increase by 0.5 J/cm^2 every treatment up to 2 J/cm^2 as tolerated. Consult the attending physician if burning has occurred. Higher doses of UVA must be ordered by the physician.

15. The frequency of bath PUVA treatments for the diagnosis of psoriasis is 1 or 2 times a week unless otherwise ordered by a physician. If more than 2 times a week has been ordered, then special instructions as to the advancement of the dose of UVA light must accompany the request.

16. If the skin is red, the phototherapist will contact the attending physician who will make the decision for adjustment in the treatment for that day. If the skin is a light pink color, the phototherapist should keep the dose the same as the previously delivered treatment dose.

17. If subsequent treatments occur at intervals longer than 3 days, the following guidelines will be used:

1 week	Keep the dose the same.
2 weeks	Decrease the dose by 50%.
3 weeks	Start over.

18. Follow steps 3–13 previously.

PSORALEN LOTION PLUS ULTRAVIOLET A (PAINT PUVA)

PATIENT INSTRUCTIONS

1. All patients designated for paint PUVA will have the routine introduction to the PTC facility.

2. All patients designated for paint PUVA will have the basic introduction to phototherapy equipment and safety procedures.

3. Reinforcement of the need for eye protection for all patients and covering of the genital area in males is required if total body PUVA is to be done.

4. Patients receiving paint PUVA will be instructed to apply the psoralen lotion applied with a cotton-tipped applicator to the areas to be treated for 30 minutes immediately preceding the delivery of the UVA light. This area is to be protected or covered with protective fabric if done outside the confines of the treatment center.

5. All patients receiving paint PUVA must wear protective clothing or sun-block containing both UVA or UVB sunscreen after washing the treated areas following the delivery of UVA light.

6. A handheld timer, set by the phototherapy technician, will be given to the patient to have with them during each phototherapy session. The time will correspond with the amount of time calculated for their dose of UVA for that treatment.

7. Instruct patients to complete the treatment session when the lights have gone out or within 10 seconds of the alarm of the safety (handheld) timer.

8. A list of current medications will be placed in the patient's chart and reviewed by the phototherapist. Questions concerning the current medications will be addressed by the attending physician.

9. All patients will be told of the possible complications of paint PUVA phototherapy specifically including

    a. Sunburn reaction
    b. Corneal burn if the eyes are unprotected
    c. Cataract formation if the eyes are unprotected
    d. Photoallergic dermatitis (including drug reaction)
    e. Freckling of the skin
    f. Aging of the skin
    g. Increase in risk of skin cancers including melanoma

10. Patients will be told that additional sun exposure should be avoided on the days they receive paint PUVA. The patients should be told that UVA light is transmitted through window and auto glass.

11. All patients will be given the brochure on PUVA phototherapy from the National Psoriasis Foundation.

PROTOCOL

1. Obtain a signed consent form after the patient has been given the tour of the PTC and basic phototherapy education concerning PUVA phototherapy. The patient should be given time for questions.

2. A lotion containing 0.01% of 8-methoxypsoralen should be prescribed to the patient for their use. The compounding of this lotion should be done by a pharmacist. The 8-methoxypsoralen may also be prepared in an ointment base using Aquaphor or a Vaseline base. The concentration for the ointment-based psoralen preparation is 0.1% of 8-methoxypsoralen.

3. Apply the psoralen lotion to the involved areas with a cotton-tipped applicator. Only apply the psoralen to the sites to be treated. This is best done in the treatment center with the aid of a technician, especially in hard-to-reach areas. However, the lotion may be applied by the patient prior to the time of the scheduled treatment with UVA. The duration of the pretreatment with the topical psoralen should be 30 minutes. The delivery of the dose of UVA light should follow the 30-minute pretreatment period. If desired, uninvolved areas adjacent to the treated sites can be wrapped with multiple layers of cloth to provide protection from UVA light.

4. The initial dose of UVA for paint PUVA is 0.5 J/cm^2 for all skin types.

5. The irradiance (mW/cm^2) of the UVA light unit should be recorded on a once-a-month basis using the standard method of the manufacturer of the phototherapy unit. Record this irradiance on the phototherapy record sheet or keep an irradiance logbook for the equipment used in patient care.

6. The manual method for calculation of the time (seconds) to set the UV control panel to deliver the dose from #4 is the following equation: (The measurement of the irradiance can be obtained from the logbook kept on a weekly basis.)

$$\text{Time (seconds)} = \text{Dose (mJ/cm}^2) \div \text{Irradiance (mW/cm}^2)$$

7. The duration of a treatment or total dose of UV light to be delivered can often be calculated by the UV light unit by following the manufacturer's instructions in the operations manual and inputting the correct information on the control panel prior to the delivery of the treatment.

8. Set the time (or dose) on the control panel of the UV light unit and on the additional safety timer kept in the light unit or by the technician. In some phototherapy units, the session duration is dependent on the dose measured by an internal photometer, and the time must be estimated by the technician.

9. Verify that the UV light unit is set on UVA.

10. Have the patient put on protective glasses during the phototherapy treatment session.

11. Start the treatment.

12. After the UVA treatment is given, the patient must thoroughly wash the treated areas to remove any medication residue on the surface of the skin. Sunblock (UVA/B) is provided for the patient to apply as a precautionary measure to avoid additional UV exposure that day.

13. Instruct the patient to avoid excessive sunlight for the remainder of the day. A burn may not show up until 48 hours after treatment. Treatments are not usually given on 2 consecutive days. This allows the nurse to observe accurately for erythema.

14. Advise the patient that areas around the vitiligo may become darker in color during treatment.

15. Each patient should be seen by the attending physician 4 weeks after the first treatment, and then every 6–8 weeks during treatment. The patient should be seen immediately by a physician if any problems with treatment arise.

SUBSEQUENT TREATMENTS

16. Increase by 0.5 J/cm^2 every treatment as tolerated up to 2 J/cm^2. Consult the attending physician if burning has occurred. Higher doses of UVA must be ordered by the physician.

17. The frequency of paint PUVA treatments for the diagnosis of vitiligo is 1–2 times a week unless otherwise ordered by a physician. If more than 2 times a week has been ordered, then special instructions as to the advancement of the dose of UVA light must accompany the request.

18. If the skin is red, the phototherapist will contact the attending physician who will make the decision for adjustment in the treatment for that day. If the skin is a light pink color, the phototherapist should keep the dose the same as the previously delivered treatment dose.

19. If subsequent treatments occur at intervals longer than 3 days, the following guidelines will be used:

1 week	Keep the dose the same.
2 weeks	Decrease the dose by 50%.
3 weeks	Start over.

20. Follow steps 3–15 previously.

Atopic Dermatitis

ULTRAVIOLET B PHOTOTHERAPY

PATIENT INSTRUCTIONS

1. All patients designated for the ultraviolet B (UVB) protocol will have the routine introduction to the Phototherapy Treatment Center (PTC) facility.

2. All patients designated for the UVB protocol will have the basic introduction to phototherapy equipment and safety procedures.

3. Reinforcement of the need for eye protection for all patients and covering of the genital area in males is required.

4. Patients are to stand in the center of the light cabinet with their arms at rest. A step stool may be used for the patients to stand on when recommended by the physician.

5. A hand-held timer will be set by the phototherapy technician for each treatment session. The time will correspond to the estimated time of the treatment session duration, and the timer will either be given to the patients to have with them during the treatment session or be kept by the technician during the treatment. The time will correspond with the amount of time calculated for their dose of UVB for that treatment.

6. Instruct patients to come out of the light box when the lights have gone out or within 10 seconds of the alarm of the safety (hand-held) timer. Inform patients that the light-box doors are not locked and demonstrate their operation.

7. The list of current medications will be placed in the patient chart and reviewed by the phototherapist. Questions concerning the current medications will be addressed by the attending physicians.

8. All patients will be told of the possible complications of UVB phototherapy specifically including

    a. Sunburn reaction
    b. Corneal burn if the eyes are unprotected
    c. Photoallergic dermatitis (including drug reaction)
    d. Freckling of the skin
    e. Aging of the skin
    f. Possible increase in risk of skin cancers

9. Patients will be told that additional unprotected sun exposure should be avoided on the days they receive UVB. Sunblock (SPF 15) should be used on any sun-exposed areas for the remainder of that day.

10. All patients will be given the brochure on UVB phototherapy from the National Psoriasis Foundation.

PROTOCOL

1. Obtain a signed consent form after the patient has been given the tour of the PTC and basic phototherapy education concerning UVB phototherapy. The patient should be given time for questions.

2. Have the patient undress completely. Male patients should wear an athletic supporter unless otherwise directed or permitted by the attending physician.

3. Eye protection in the form of UV goggles must be worn by all patients when inside the phototherapy unit.

4. The irradiance (mW/cm^2) of the UVB light inside the unit should be recorded on a once-a-month basis using the standard method of the manufacturer of the phototherapy unit. Record this irradiance on the phototherapy record sheet or keep an irradiance logbook for the equipment used in patient care.

5. Determine the initial UVB dose (mJ/cm^2) according to the patient's skin type as classified by the physician. See Appendix for definitions of skin types.

Skin Type	Initial UVB Dose (mJ/cm^2)
Type I	10
Type II	10
Type III	20
Type IV	20
Type V	30
Type VI	30

6. The manual method for calculation of the time (seconds) to set the UVB control panel to deliver the dose from #5 is the following equation: (The measurement of the irradiance can be obtained from the logbook kept on a weekly basis.)

$$\text{Time (seconds)} = \text{Dose } (mJ/cm^2) \div \text{Irradiance } (mW/cm^2)$$

7. The duration of a treatment or total dose of UVB to be delivered can often be calculated by the ultraviolet light unit by following the manufacturer's instructions in the operations manual and inputting the correct information on the control panel prior to the delivery of the treatment.

8. Set the time (or dose) on the control panel of the ultraviolet light unit and on the additional safety timer kept in the light unit or by the technician. In some phototherapy units, the session duration is dependent on the dose measured by an internal photometer, and the time must be estimated by the technician.

9. Verify that the ultraviolet light unit is set on UVB.

10. Turn on the fan and have the patient stand in the center of the ultraviolet light unit with their arms at rest. Double-check that they are wearing UV goggles as eye protection.

11. Instruct the patient to come out of the ultraviolet light box when the lights go out or if they become uncomfortable during the treatment either from burning or stinging of the skin. Inform the patient that the light-box doors are not locked.

12. Start the treatment.

SUBSEQUENT TREATMENTS

13. The frequency of UVB light treatments for the diagnosis of atopic dermatitis is 3 times a week unless otherwise ordered by a physician. If less than 2 times a week has been ordered by a physician, then special instructions for the advancement of the dose of UVB light must accompany the request.

14. On subsequent visits, the patient will be asked about redness, light pink color, and tenderness of the skin the previous night, and this information will be put into the phototherapy record.

15. If the skin is red, the phototherapy technician will ask that the patient be seen by the attending physician who will make the decision for adjustment in the UVB treatment. If the skin is a light pink color, the phototherapist should keep the dose the same as the previously delivered treatment dose.

16. Increase the dose (mJ/cm^2) of the UVB light by the amount mentioned down and add it to the previous dose delivered to the patient if the treatment has been within 3 days:

Skin Type	Amount of UVB Increase (mJ/cm^2)
Type I	5
Type II	5
Type III	10
Type IV	10
Type V	20
Type VI	20

17. For subsequent treatments, if the time between treatments has been

4–7 days	Keep the dose the same.
1–2 weeks	Decrease the dose by 50%.
2–3 weeks	Decrease the dose by 75%.
3 or more weeks	Start over.

18. Follow steps 6–12 aforementioned.

19. The dose and frequency of UVB light will be adjusted by the physician according to the response to therapy. The dose of UVB for the diagnosis of atopic dermatitis should not exceed the following guidelines for each skin type:

Skin Type	UVB Dose (mJ/cm^2)
Type I	50
Type II	50
Type III	100
Type IV	100
Type V	200
Type VI	200

COMBINATION ULTRAVIOLET A/B PHOTOTHERAPY

PATIENT INSTRUCTIONS

1. All patients designated for the ultraviolet A/B (UVA/B) protocol for atopic dermatitis will have the routine introduction to the PTC facility.

2. All patients designated for the UVA/B protocol will have the basic introduction to phototherapy equipment and safety procedures.

3. Reinforcement of the need for eye protection for all patients and covering of the genital area in males is required.

4. Patients are to stand in the center of the light cabinet with their arms at rest. A step stool may be used for the patients to stand on when recommended by the physician.

5. A hand-held timer will be set by the phototherapy technician for each treatment session. The time will correspond to the estimated time of the treatment session duration for the UVB segment of the treatment, and the timer will either be given to the patient to have with them during the treatment session or be kept by the technician during the treatment. The time will correspond with the amount of time calculated for their dose of UVB for that treatment.

6. Instruct patients to come out of the light box if the UVB lights have not gone out or within 10 seconds of the alarm of the safety (hand-held) timer. There will be a longer duration of the UVA lights, which will complete the treatment. Inform patients that the light-box doors are not locked and demonstrate their operation.

7. The list of current medications will be placed in the patient chart and reviewed by the phototherapist. Questions concerning the current medications will be addressed by the attending physician.

8. All patients will be told of the possible complications of UV phototherapy specifically including

    a. Sunburn reaction
    b. Corneal burn if the eyes are unprotected
    c. Photoallergic dermatitis (including drug reaction)
    d. Freckling of the skin
    e. Aging of the skin
    f. Increase in risk of skin cancers

9. Patients will be told that additional unprotected sun exposure should be avoided the days they receive UVB. Sunblock (SPF 15) should be used on any sun-exposed areas for the remainder of that day.

10. All patients will be given the brochure on UVB phototherapy from the National Psoriasis Foundation.

PROTOCOL

1. Obtain a signed consent form after the patient has been given the tour of the PTC and basic phototherapy education concerning phototherapy. The patient should be given time for questions.

2. Have the patient undress completely. Male patients should wear an athletic supporter unless otherwise directed or permitted by the attending physician.

3. Eye protection in the form of UV goggles must be worn by all patients when inside the phototherapy unit.

4. The irradiance (mW/cm^2) of the UVA and UVB light inside the unit should be recorded on a once-a-month basis using the standard method of the manufacturer of the phototherapy unit. Record this irradiance on the phototherapy record sheet or keep an irradiance logbook for the equipment used in patient care.

5. Determine the initial UVB and UVA dose according to the patient's skin type as classified by the physician. See Appendix for definitions of skin types.

Skin Type	UVB Dose (mJ/cm^2)	UVA Dose (J/cm^2)
Type I	10	2
Type II	10	2
Type III	20	4
Type IV	20	4
Type V	30	6
Type VI	30	6

6. The manual method for calculation of the time (seconds) to set the UVA and UVB control panels to deliver the dose from #5 is the following equation: (The measurement of the irradiance can be obtained from the logbook kept on a weekly basis.)

$$\text{Time (seconds)} = \text{Dose (mJ/cm}^2) \div \text{Irradiance (mW/cm}^2)$$

7. The duration of a treatment or total dose of UV light to be delivered can often be calculated by the ultraviolet light unit by following the manufacturer's instructions in the operation manual and inputting the correct information on the control panel prior to the delivery of the treatment.

8. Set the time (or dose) on the control panel of the ultraviolet light unit for both the UVA and UVB panels and on the additional safety timer, which will correspond to the UVB segment of the treatment and be kept in the light unit or by the technician. In some phototherapy units, the session duration is dependent on the dose measured by an internal photometer, and the time must be estimated by the technician.

9. Verify that the ultraviolet light unit is set on UVB for the correct dose and UVA for the correct dose.

10. Turn on the fan and have the patient stand in the center of the ultraviolet light unit with their arms at rest. Double-check that they are wearing UV goggles as eye protection.

11. Instruct the patient to come out of the ultraviolet light box when the lights go out or if they become uncomfortable during the treatment either from burning or stinging of the skin. Inform the patient that the light-box doors are not locked.

12. Start the treatment.

SUBSEQUENT TREATMENTS

13. The frequency of UVA/B light treatments for the diagnosis of atopic dermatitis is 3 times a week unless otherwise ordered by a physician. If less than 2 times a week has been ordered, then special instructions as to the advancement of the dose of UVA/B light must accompany the request.

14. On subsequent visits, the patient will be asked about redness, light pink color, and tenderness of the skin the previous night, and this information will be put into the phototherapy record.

15. If the skin is red, the phototherapist will ask that the patient be seen by the attending physician who will make the decision for adjustment in the UVA/B treatment. If the skin is a light pink color, the phototherapist should keep the dose the same as the previously delivered treatment dose.

16. Increase the dose of the UVA/B light by the amount as follows and add it to the previous dose delivered to the patient if the treatment has been within 3 days:

Skin Type	UVB Dose (mJ/cm²)	UVA Dose (J/cm²)
Type I	5	1
Type II	5	1
Type III	10	1
Type IV	10	1
Type V	20	1
Type VI	20	1

17. For subsequent treatments, if the time between treatments has been greater than 3 days, follow the guidelines given down:

4–7 days	Keep the dose the same.
1–2 weeks	Decrease the dose by 50%.
2–3 weeks	Decrease the dose by 75%.
3 or more weeks	Start over.

18. The dose and frequency of UVB light will be adjusted by the physician according to the response to therapy. The dose of UVB for the diagnosis of atopic dermatitis should not exceed the following guidelines for each skin type:

Skin Type	Maximum UVB Dose (mJ/cm²)	Maximum UVA Dose (J/cm²)
Type I	50	10
Type II	50	10
Type III	100	20
Type IV	100	20
Type V	200	40
Type VI	200	40

19. Follow steps 6–12 aforementioned.

NARROWBAND ULTRAVIOLET B PHOTOTHERAPY

PATIENT INSTRUCTIONS

1. All patients designated for the narrowband ultraviolet B (NBUVB) protocol for atopic dermatitis will have the routine introduction to the PTC facility.

2. All patients designated for the NBUVB protocol will have the basic introduction to phototherapy equipment and safety procedures.

3. Reinforcement of the need for eye protection for all patients and covering of the genital area in males is required.

4. Patients are to stand in the center of the light cabinet with their arms at rest. A step stool may be used for the patients to stand on when recommended by the physician.

5. A hand-held timer will be set by the phototherapy technician for each treatment session. The time will correspond to the estimated time of the treatment session duration, and the timer will either be given to the patients to have with them during the treatment session or be kept by the technician during the treatment. The time will correspond with the amount of time calculated for their dose of NBUVB for that treatment.

6. Instruct patients to come out of the light box when the lights have gone out or within 10 seconds of the alarm of the safety (hand-held) timer. Inform patients that the light-box doors are not locked and demonstrate their operation.

7. The list of current medications will be placed in the patient chart and reviewed by the phototherapist. Questions concerning the current medications will be addressed by the attending physicians.

8. All patients will be told of the possible complications of NBUVB phototherapy specifically including

   a. Sunburn reaction
   b. Corneal burn if the eyes are unprotected
   c. Photoallergic dermatitis (including drug reaction)
   d. Freckling of the skin
   e. Aging of the skin
   f. Possible increase in risk of skin cancers

9. Patients will be told that additional unprotected sun exposure should be avoided on the days they receive NBUVB. Sunblock (SPF 15) should be used on any sun-exposed areas for the remainder of that day.

10. All patients will be given the brochure on UVB phototherapy from the National Psoriasis Foundation.

PROTOCOL

1. Obtain a signed consent form after the patient has been given the tour of the PTC and basic phototherapy education concerning NBUVB phototherapy. The patient should be given time for questions.

2. Have the patient undress and expose the areas of atopic dermatitis to be treated. Male patients should wear an athletic supporter unless otherwise directed or permitted by the attending physician.

3. Eye protection in the form of UV goggles must be worn by all patients when inside the phototherapy unit.

4. The irradiance (mW/cm^2) of the NBUVB light inside the unit should be recorded on a once-a-month basis using the standard method of the manufacturer of the phototherapy unit. Record this irradiance on the phototherapy record sheet or keep an irradiance logbook for the equipment used in patient care.

5. The initial NBUVB dose (mJ/cm^2) will be the same for all patients with atopic dermatitis. It is 300 mJ/cm^2.

6. The manual method for calculation of the time (seconds) to set the NBUVB control panel to deliver the dose from #5 is the following equation: (The measurement of the irradiance can be obtained from the logbook kept on a weekly basis.)

$$\text{Time (seconds)} = \text{Dose } (mJ/cm^2) \div \text{Irradiance } (mW/cm^2)$$

7. The duration of a treatment or total dose of NBUVB to be delivered can often be calculated by the ultraviolet light unit by following the manufacturer's instructions in the operations manual and inputting the correct information on the control panel prior to the delivery of the treatment.

8. Set the time (or dose) on the control panel of the ultraviolet light unit and on the additional safety timer kept in the light unit or by the technician. In some phototherapy units, the session duration is dependent on the dose measured by an internal photometer, and the time must be estimated by the technician.

9. Verify that the ultraviolet light unit is set on NBUVB.

10. Turn on the fan and have the patient stand in the center of the ultraviolet light unit with their arms at rest. Double-check that they are wearing UV goggles as eye protection.

11. Instruct the patient to come out of the ultraviolet light box when the lights go out or if they become uncomfortable during the treatment either from burning or stinging of the skin. Inform the patient that the light-box doors are not locked.

12. Start the treatment.

SUBSEQUENT TREATMENTS

13. The frequency of NBUVB light treatments for the diagnosis of atopic dermatitis is 2 or 3 times a week unless otherwise ordered by a physician. If more than 3 times a week has been ordered by a physician, then special instructions for the advancement of the dose of NBUVB light must accompany the request.

14. On subsequent visits, the patient will be asked about redness, light pink color, and tenderness of the skin the previous night, and this information will be put into the phototherapy record.

15. If the skin is red, the phototherapy technician will ask that the patient be seen by the attending physician who will make the decision for adjustment in the NBUVB treatment. If the skin is a light pink color, the phototherapist should keep the dose the same as the previously delivered treatment dose.

16. Increase the dose (mJ/cm^2) of the NBUVB light by the amount as follows and add it to the previous dose delivered to the patient if the treatment has been within 3 days:

    Subsequent treatments—increase by 100 mJ/cm^2

17. Do not exceed 1000 mJ/cm^2 unless otherwise ordered by the physician.

18. For subsequent treatments, if the time between treatments has been

4–7 days	Keep the dose the same.
1–2 weeks	Decrease the dose by 50%.
2–3 weeks	Start over.

19. Follow steps 6–12 aforementioned.

SYSTEMIC PSORALEN PLUS ULTRAVIOLET A

PATIENT INSTRUCTIONS

1. All patients designated for psoralen plus ultraviolet A (PUVA) for atopic dermatitis will have the routine introduction to the PTC facility.

2. All patients designated for PUVA will have the basic introduction to phototherapy equipment and safety procedures.

3. Reinforcement of the need for eye protection for all patients and covering of the genital area in males is required.

4. Patients receiving systemic PUVA will be instructed to take Oxsoralen Ultra® tablets in the dose prescribed by their physician 1 hour prior to the estimated time of their arrival at the PTC. The treatment will be given between 1 hour 15 minutes and 1 hour 45 minutes after the ingestion of the medication.

5. All patients ingesting Oxsoralen Ultra must wear protective UV blocking glasses when outside, riding in a car, or next to a window from the time they take the medication and for the next 18–24 hours during daylight.

6. Patients are to stand in the center of the light cabinet with their arms at rest. A step stool may be used for the patients to stand on when recommended by the physician.

7. A hand-held timer will be set by the phototherapy technician for each treatment session. The time will correspond to the estimated time of the treatment session duration, and the timer will either be given to the patients to have with them during the treatment session or be kept by the technician during the treatment. The time will correspond with the amount of time calculated for their dose of UVA for that treatment.

8. Instruct patients to come out of the light box when the lights have gone out or within 10 seconds of the alarm of the safety (hand-held) timer. Inform patients that the light-box doors are not locked and demonstrate their operation.

9. The list of current medications will be placed in the patient chart and reviewed by the phototherapist. Questions concerning the current medications will be addressed by the attending physician.

10. All patients will be told of the possible complications of PUVA phototherapy specifically including

    a. Sunburn reaction
    b. Corneal burn if the eyes are unprotected
    c. Cataract formation if the eyes are unprotected
    d. Photoallergic dermatitis (including drug reaction)

      e.   Freckling of the skin

      f.   Aging of the skin

      g.   Increase in risk of skin cancers including melanoma

11.   Patients will be told that additional unprotected sun exposure should be avoided on the days they receive PUVA. Wide-spectrum sunblock (UVA/B) should be used on any sun-exposed areas for the remainder of that day.

12.   All patients will be given the brochure on PUVA phototherapy from the National Psoriasis Foundation.

PROTOCOL

1. Obtain a signed consent form after the patient has been given the tour of the PTC and basic phototherapy education concerning PUVA phototherapy. The patient should be given time for questions.

2. Oxsoralen Ultra (8-methoxypsoralen) is to be ingested by the patient at least 1 hour prior to arrival at the PTC. Treatments may be given anytime between 1 hour 15 minutes and 1 hour 45 minutes after ingestion.

3. Dosage of the Oxsoralen Ultra tablets is dependent on the orders of the attending physician and will vary from patient to patient. The standard dosage is 0.5–0.6 mg/kg.

4. Ask the patient at what time they ingested their medication and how many pills they ingested.

5. Have the patient undress completely unless otherwise ordered by the physician. Male patients should wear an athletic supporter unless otherwise directed or permitted by the attending physician.

6. Eye protection in the form of UV goggles must be worn by all patients when inside the phototherapy unit.

7. The irradiance (mW/cm^2) of the UVA light inside the unit should be recorded on a once-a-month basis using the standard method of the manufacturer of the phototherapy unit. Record this irradiance on the phototherapy record sheet or keep an irradiance logbook for the equipment used in patient care.

8. Determine the initial PUVA dose (J/cm^2) according to the patient's skin type as classified by the physician. See Appendix for definitions of skin types.

Skin Type	Initial UVA Dose (J/cm^2)
Type I	1
Type II	1
Type III	2
Type IV	2
Type V	3
Type VI	3

9. The manual method for calculation of the time (seconds) to set the UVA control panel to deliver the dose from #8 is the following equation: (The measurement of the irradiance can be obtained from the logbook kept on a weekly basis.)

$$\text{Time (seconds)} = \text{Dose (mJ/cm}^2) \div \text{Irradiance (mW/cm}^2)$$

10. The duration of a treatment or total dose of UVA to be delivered can often be calculated by the ultraviolet light unit by following the manufacturer's instructions in the operations manual and inputting the correct information on the control panel prior to the delivery of the treatment.

11. Set the time (or dose) on the control panel of the ultraviolet light unit and on the additional safety timer kept in the light unit or by the technician. In some phototherapy units, the session duration is dependent on the dose measured by an internal photometer and the time must be estimated by the technician.

12. Verify that the ultraviolet light unit is set on UVA.

13. Turn on the fan and have the patient stand in the center of the ultraviolet light unit with their arms at rest. Double-check that they are wearing UV goggles as eye protection.

14. Instruct the patient to come out of the ultraviolet light box when the lights go out or if they become uncomfortable during the treatment either from burning or stinging of the skin. Inform the patient that the light-box doors are not locked.

15. Start the treatment.

16. Some patients may receive localized ultraviolet light therapy to the legs or trunk as ordered by the physician.

17. An ophthalmology examination should be performed prior to and every 6 months during PUVA therapy.

18. Laboratory monitoring is done at baseline and every 6 months as necessary.

SUBSEQUENT TREATMENTS

19. The frequency of PUVA treatments for the diagnosis of atopic dermatitis is 2 or 3 times a week unless ordered by a physician. If more than 3 times a week has been ordered, then special instructions as to the advancement of the dose of UVA light must accompany the request.

20. On subsequent visits, the patient will be asked about redness, light pink color, and tenderness of the skin the previous night, and this information will be put into the phototherapy record. The patient will also be asked at what time they took the psoralen tablets.

21. If the skin is red, the phototherapist will ask that the patient be seen by the attending physician who will make the decision for adjustment in the treatment for that day. If the skin is a light pink color, the phototherapist should keep the dose the same as the previously delivered treatment dose.

22. Increase the dose (J/cm^2) of the UVA light by the amount as follows and add it to the previous dose delivered to the patient if the treatment has been within 3 days:

Skin Type	Amount of UVA Increase (J/cm^2)
Type I	0.5
Type II	0.5
Type III	1.0
Type IV	1.0
Type V	1.5
Type VI	1.5

23. Do not exceed 20 J/cm^2 unless ordered by a physician.

24. If subsequent treatments occur at intervals longer than 3 days, the following guidelines will be used:

1 week	Keep the dose the same.
2 weeks	Decrease the dose by 25%–50%.
3 weeks	Decrease the dose by 50%–75%.
4 weeks	Start over.

25. Follow steps 4–15 aforementioned.

HYDROSOUND BATH

PATIENT INSTRUCTIONS

1. Show the patients the hydrosound bath room.

2. Explain to the patient how to use emergency call light by pulling on the wallmounted cord within reach of the tub.

3. The patient will be told they may undress in the bath area.

4. Patients must be told they will be in the tub for 15 minutes unless they have uncomfortable ringing in their ears or stinging of their skin.

5. Instruct male patients to wear swim trunks or an athletic supporter.

6. Patients will be asked to enter the tub with assistance. If there is any difficulty stepping into the tub the patient lift is available for their use.

Protocol

1. Fill the tank with water (95°F) above the ultrasound plate. Place a rubber mat in the bottom of the tub.

2. Add hydrosound water conditioner to the tub water by pumping the measured dispenser 3 times into the tub.

3. Turn the timer to 20 minutes with an intensity of 100, to de-gas the water as per the instructions from the manufacturer.

4. Assist the patient into the tub; use the patient lift if the patient has any difficulty stepping into the tub. Patients must be able to stand unassisted to be able to use the patient lift and to be considered for hydrosound therapy.

5. Turn the hydrosound timer on. The standard length of time for a hydrosound bath is 15 minutes. The time may be adjusted as per physician orders.

6. Set the timer on the hydrosound control panel to 15 minutes.

7. Leave the intensity at 100 unless the patient complains of ringing in the ears or stinging on the skin. The intensity may then be adjusted to 80. If the ringing in the ears or stinging is still uncomfortable to the patient, then the treatment is to be stopped and the physician notified.

8. The patients will be attended by PTC personnel either in the room or in the hallway of the bath facility with the door open throughout the duration of the hydrosound bath.

9. Assist the patient out of tub at the end of the treatment.

10. Drain the water from the tub.

11. Clean the tub per manufacturer's instructions with disinfectant solution, using a cloth to wipe down the tub. Let it stand for 2 minutes, then rinse.

Pruritus

ULTRAVIOLET B PHOTOTHERAPY

PATIENT INSTRUCTIONS

1. All patients designated for the ultraviolet B (UVB) protocol will have the routine introduction to the Phototherapy Treatment Center (PTC) facility.

2. All patients designated for the UVB protocol will have the basic introduction to phototherapy equipment and safety procedures.

3. Reinforcement of the need for eye protection for all patients and covering of the genital area in males is required.

4. Patients are to stand in the center of the light cabinet with their arms at rest. A step stool may be used for the patients to stand on when recommended by the physician.

5. A hand-held timer will be set by the phototherapy technician for each treatment session. The time will correspond to the estimated time of the treatment session duration, and the timer will either be given to the patients to have with them during the treatment session or be kept by the technician during the treatment. The time will correspond with the amount of time calculated for their dose of UVB for that treatment.

6. Instruct patients to come out of the light box when the lights have gone out or within 10 seconds of the alarm of the safety (hand-held) timer. Inform patients that the light-box doors are not locked and demonstrate their operation.

7. The list of current medications will be placed in the patient chart and reviewed by the phototherapist. Questions concerning the current medications will be addressed by the attending physician.

8. All patients will be told of the possible complications of UVB phototherapy specifically including

    a. Sunburn reaction
    b. Corneal burn if the eyes are unprotected
    c. Photoallergic dermatitis (including drug reaction)
    d. Freckling of the skin
    e. Aging of the skin
    f. Possible increase in risk of skin cancers

9. Patients will be told that additional unprotected sun exposure should be avoided on the days they receive UVB. Sunblock (SPF 15) should be used on any sun-exposed areas for the remainder of that day.

10. All patients will be given the brochure on UVB phototherapy from the National Psoriasis Foundation.

PROTOCOL

1. Obtain a signed consent form after the patient has been given the tour of the PTC and basic phototherapy education concerning UVB phototherapy. The patient should be given time for questions.

2. Have the patient undress completely. Male patients should wear an athletic supporter unless otherwise directed or permitted by the attending physician.

3. Eye protection in the form of UV goggles must be worn by all patients when inside the phototherapy unit.

4. The irradiance (mW/cm^2) of the UVB light inside the unit should be recorded on a once-a-month basis using the standard method of the manufacturer of the phototherapy unit. Record this irradiance on the phototherapy record sheet or keep an irradiance logbook for the equipment used in the patient care.

5. Determine the initial UVB dose (mJ/cm^2) according to the patient's skin type as classified by the physician. See Appendix for definitions of skin types.

Skin Type	Initial UVB Dose (mJ/cm^2)
Type I	10
Type II	10
Type III	20
Type IV	20
Type V	30
Type VI	30

6. The manual method for calculation of the time (seconds) to set the UVB control panel to deliver the dose from #5 is the following equation: (The measurement of the irradiance can be obtained from the logbook kept on a weekly basis.)

$$\text{Time (seconds)} = \text{Dose (mJ/cm}^2) \div \text{Irradiance (mW/cm}^2)$$

7. The duration of a treatment or total dose of UVB to be delivered can often be calculated by the ultraviolet light unit by following the manufacturer's instructions in the operations manual and inputting the correct information on the control panel prior to the delivery of the treatment.

8. Set the time (or dose) on the control panel of the ultraviolet light unit and on the additional safety timer kept in the light unit or by the technician. In some phototherapy units, the session duration is dependent on the dose measured by an internal photometer, and the time must be estimated by the technician.

9. Verify that the ultraviolet light unit is set on UVB.

10. Turn on the fan and have the patient stand in the center of the ultraviolet light unit with their arms at rest. Double-check that they are wearing UV goggles as eye protection.

11. Instruct the patient to come out of the ultraviolet light box when the lights go out or if they become uncomfortable during the treatment either from burning or stinging of the skin. Inform the patient that the light-box doors are not locked.

12. Start the treatment.

SUBSEQUENT TREATMENTS

13. The frequency of UVB light treatments for the diagnosis of pruritus is 2 or 3 times a week unless otherwise ordered by a physician. If less than 2 times a week has been ordered, then special instructions for the advancement of the dose of UVB light must accompany the request.

14. On subsequent visits, the patient will be asked about redness, light pink color, and tenderness of the skin the previous night, and this information will be put into the phototherapy record.

15. If the skin is red, the phototherapy technician will ask that the patient be seen by the attending physician who will make the decision for adjustment in the UVB treatment. If the skin is a light pink color, the phototherapist should keep the dose the same as the previously delivered treatment dose.

16. Increase the dose (mJ/cm^2) of the UVB light by the amount given down and add it to the previous dose delivered to the patient if the treatment has been within 3 days:

Skin Type	Increase in UVB Dose (mJ/cm^2)
Type I	5
Type II	5
Type III	10
Type IV	10
Type V	20
Type VI	20

17. For subsequent treatments, if the time between treatments has been

4–7 days	Keep the dose the same.
1–2 weeks	Decrease the dose by 50%.
2–3 weeks	Decrease the dose by 75%.
3 or more weeks	Start over.

18. The dose and frequency of UVB light will be adjusted by the physician according to the response to therapy. The dose of UVB for the diagnosis of pruritus should not exceed the following guidelines for each skin type:

Skin Type	UVB Dose (mJ/cm^2)
Type I	50
Type II	50
Type III	100
Type IV	100
Type V	200
Type VI	200

19. Follow steps 6–12 aforementioned.

COMBINATION ULTRAVIOLET A/B PHOTOTHERAPY

PATIENT INSTRUCTIONS

1. All patients designated for the ultraviolet A/B (UVA/B) protocol for pruritus will have the routine introduction to the PTC facility.

2. All patients designated for the UVA/B protocol will have the basic introduction to phototherapy equipment and safety procedures.

3. Reinforcement of the need for eye protection for all patients and covering of the genital area in males is required.

4. Patients are to stand in the center of the light cabinet with their arms at rest. A step stool may be used for the patients to stand on when recommended by the physician.

5. A hand-held timer will be set by the phototherapy technician for each treatment session. The time will correspond to the estimated time of the treatment session duration, and the timer will either be given to the patients to have with them during the treatment session or be kept by the technician during the treatment. The time will correspond with the amount of time calculated for their dose of UVA/B for that treatment.

6. Instruct patients to come out of the light box when the lights have gone out or within 10 seconds of the alarm of the safety (hand-held) timer. Inform patients that the light-box doors are not locked and demonstrate their operation.

7. The list of current medications will be placed on the patient chart and reviewed by the phototherapist. Questions concerning current medications will be addressed by the attending physician.

8. All patients will be told of the possible complications of UV phototherapy specifically including

    a. Sunburn reaction
    b. Corneal burn if the eyes are unprotected
    c. Photoallergic dermatitis (including drug reaction)
    d. Freckling of the skin
    e. Aging of the skin
    f. Possible increase in risk of skin cancers

9. Patients will be told that additional unprotected sun exposure should be avoided on the days they receive UVA/B. Sunblock (SPF 15) should be used on any sun-exposed areas for the remainder of that day.

10. All patients will be given the brochure on UVB phototherapy from the National Psoriasis Foundation.

PROTOCOL

1. Obtain a signed consent form after the patient has been given the tour of the PTC and basic phototherapy education concerning phototherapy. The patient should be given time for questions.

2. Have the patient undress completely. Male patients should wear an athletic supporter unless otherwise directed or permitted by the attending physician.

3. Eye protection in the form of UV goggles must be worn by all patients when inside the phototherapy unit.

4. The irradiance (mW/cm^2) of the UVA and UVB light inside the unit should be recorded on a once-a-month basis using the standard method of the manufacturer of the phototherapy unit. Record this irradiance on the phototherapy record sheet or keep an irradiance logbook for the equipment used in patient care.

5. Determine the initial UVB and UVA dose according to the patient's skin type as classified by the physician. See Appendix for definitions of skin types.

Skin Type	UVB Dose (mJ/cm^2)	UVA Dose (J/cm^2)
Type I	10	2
Type II	10	2
Type III	20	4
Type IV	20	4
Type V	30	6
Type VI	30	6

6. The manual method for calculation of the time (seconds) to set the UVA/B control panel to deliver the dose from #5 is the following equation: (The measurement of the irradiance can be obtained from the logbook kept on a weekly basis.)

$$\text{Time (seconds)} = \text{Dose (mJ/cm}^2） \div \text{Irradiance (mW/cm}^2)$$

7. The duration of a treatment or total dose of UVA/B to be delivered can often be calculated by the ultraviolet light unit by following the manufacturer's instructions in the operations manual and inputting the correct information on the control panel prior to the delivery of the treatment.

8. Set the time (or dose) on the control panel of the ultraviolet light unit and on the additional safety timer kept in the light unit or by the technician. In some phototherapy units, the session duration is dependent on the dose measured by an internal photometer, and the time must be estimated by the technician.

9. Verify that the ultraviolet light unit is set on the correct dose for UVB and the correct dose for UVA.

10. Turn on the fan and have the patient stand in the center of the ultraviolet light unit with their arms at rest. Double-check that they are wearing UV goggles as eye protection.

11. Instruct the patient to come out of the ultraviolet light box when the lights go out or if they become uncomfortable during the treatment either from burning or stinging of the skin. Inform the patient that the light-box doors are not locked.

12. Start the treatment.

SUBSEQUENT TREATMENTS

13. The frequency of UVA/B light treatments for the diagnosis of pruritus is 3 times a week unless otherwise ordered by a physician. If less than 2 times a week has been ordered, then special instructions as to the advancement of the dose of UVA/B light must accompany the request.

14. On subsequent visits, the patient will be asked about redness, light pink color, and tenderness of the skin the previous night, and this information will be put into the phototherapy record.

15. If the skin is red, the phototherapist will ask that the patient be seen by the attending physician who will make the decision for adjustment in the UVA/B treatment. If the skin is a light pink color, the phototherapist should keep the dose the same as the previously delivered treatment dose.

16. Increase the dose of the UVA/B light by the amount given down and add it to the previous dose delivered to the patient if the treatment has been within 3 days:

Skin Type	UVB Dose (mJ/cm^2)	UVA Dose (J/cm^2)
Type I	5	1
Type II	5	1
Type III	10	1
Type IV	10	1
Type V	20	1
Type VI	20	1

17. For subsequent treatments, if the time between treatments has been greater than 3 days, follow the guideline given down:

4–7 days	Keep the dose the same.
1–2 weeks	Decrease the dose by 50%.
2–3 weeks	Decrease the dose by 75%.
3 or more weeks	Start over.

18. The dose and frequency of UVA/UVB light will be adjusted by the physician according to the response to therapy. The dose of UVB for the diagnosis of pruritus should not exceed the following guidelines for each skin type:

Skin Type	UVB Dose (mJ/cm²)	UVA Dose (J/cm²)
Type I	50	10
Type II	50	10
Type III	100	20
Type IV	100	20
Type V	200	40
Type VI	200	40

19. Follow steps 6–12 aforementioned.

NARROWBAND ULTRAVIOLET B PHOTOTHERAPY

PATIENT INSTRUCTIONS

1. All patients designated for the narrowband ultraviolet B (NBUVB) proto-col for pruritus will have the routine introduction to the PTC facility.

2. All patients designated for the NBUVB protocol will have the basic intro-duction to phototherapy equipment and safety procedures.

3. Reinforcement of the need for eye protection for all patients and covering of the genital area in males is required.

4. Patients are to stand in the center of the light cabinet with their arms at rest. A step stool may be used for the patients to stand on when recom-mended by the physician.

5. A hand-held timer will be set by the phototherapy technician for each treatment session. The time will correspond to the estimated time of the treatment session duration, and the timer will either be given to the patient to have with them during the treatment session or be kept by the techni-cian during the treatment. The time will correspond with the amount of time calculated for their dose of NBUVB for that treatment.

6. Instruct patients to come out of the light box when the lights have gone out or within 10 seconds of the alarm of the safety (hand-held) timer. Inform patients that the light-box doors are not locked and demonstrate their operation.

7. The list of current medications will be placed in the patient chart and reviewed by the phototherapist. Questions concerning the current medi-cations will be addressed by the attending physician.

8. All patients will be told of the possible complications of NBUVB photo-therapy specifically including

    a. Sunburn reaction
    b. Corneal burn if the eyes are unprotected
    c. Photoallergic dermatitis (including drug reaction)
    d. Freckling of the skin
    e. Aging of the skin
    f. Possible increase in risk of skin cancers

9. Patients will be told that additional unprotected sun exposure should be avoided the days they receive NBUVB. Sunblock (SPF 15) should be used on any sun-exposed areas for the remainder of that day.

10. All patients will be given the brochure on phototherapy from the National Psoriasis Foundation.

PROTOCOL

1. Obtain a signed consent form after the patient has been given the tour of the PTC and basic phototherapy education concerning NBUVB phototherapy. The patient should be given time for questions.

2. Have the patient undress. Male patients should wear an athletic supporter unless otherwise directed or permitted by the attending physician.

3. Eye protection in the form of UV goggles must be worn by all patients when inside the phototherapy unit.

4. The irradiance (mW/cm^2) of the NBUVB light inside the unit should be recorded on a once-a-month basis using the standard method of the manufacturer of the phototherapy unit. Record this irradiance on the phototherapy record sheet or keep an irradiance logbook for the equipment used in patient care.

5. The initial NBUVB dose (mJ/cm^2) will be the same for all patients with pruritus. It is 300 mJ/cm^2.

6. The manual method for calculation of the time (seconds) to set the NBUVB control panel to deliver the dose from #5 is the following equation: (The measurement of the irradiance can be obtained from the logbook kept on a weekly basis.)

$$\text{Time (seconds)} = \text{Dose (mJ/cm}^2) \div \text{Irradiance (mW/cm}^2)$$

7. The duration of a treatment or total dose of NBUVB to be delivered can often be calculated by the ultraviolet light unit by following the manufacturer's instructions in the operations manual and inputting the correct information on the control panel prior to the delivery of the treatment.

8. Set the time (or dose) on the control panel of the ultraviolet light unit and on the additional safety timer kept in the light unit or by the technician. In some phototherapy units, the session duration is dependent on the dose measured by an internal photometer, and the time must be estimated by the technician.

9. Verify that the ultraviolet light unit is set on NBUVB.

10. Turn on the fan and have the patient stand in the center of the ultraviolet light unit with their arms at rest. Double-check that they are wearing UV goggles as eye protection.

11. Instruct the patient to come out of the ultraviolet light box when the lights go out or if they become uncomfortable during the treatment either from burning or stinging of the skin. Inform the patient that the light-box doors are not locked.

12. Start the treatment.

SUBSEQUENT TREATMENTS

13.   The frequency of NBUVB light treatments for the diagnosis of pruritus is 2 or 3 times a week unless otherwise ordered by a physician. If more than 3 times a week has been ordered, then special instructions for the advancement of the dose of NBUVB light must accompany the request.

14.   On subsequent visits, the patient will be asked about redness, light pink color, and tenderness of the skin the previous night, and this information will be put into the phototherapy record.

15.   If the skin is red, the phototherapy technician will ask that the patient be seen by the attending physician who will make the decision for adjustment in the NBUVB treatment. If the skin is a light pink color, the phototherapist should keep the dose the same as the previously delivered treatment dose.

16.   Increase the dose (mJ/cm^2) of the NBUVB light by the amount given down and add it to the previous dose delivered to the patient if the treatment has been within 3 days.

Subsequent treatments—increase by 100 mJ/cm^2

17.   Do not exceed 1000 mJ/cm^2 unless otherwise ordered by the physician.

18.   For subsequent treatments, if the time between treatments has been

4–7 days	Keep the dose the same.
1–2 weeks	Decrease the dose by 50%.
2–3 weeks	Start over.

19.   Follow steps 6–12 aforementioned.

Cutaneous T-Cell Lymphoma

ULTRAVIOLET B PHOTOTHERAPY

PATIENT INSTRUCTIONS

1. All patients designated for the ultraviolet B (UVB) protocol will have the routine introduction to the Phototherapy Treatment Center (PTC) facility.

2. All patients designated for the UVB protocol will have the basic introduction to phototherapy equipment and safety procedures.

3. Reinforcement of the need for eye protection for all patients and covering of the genital area in males is required.

4. Patients are to stand in the center of the light cabinet with their arms at rest. A step stool may be used for the patients to stand on when recommended by the physician.

5. A hand-held timer will be set by the phototherapy technician for each treatment session. The time will correspond to the estimated time of the treatment session duration, and the timer will either be given to the patients to have with them during the treatment session or be kept by the technician during the treatment. The time will correspond with the amount of time calculated for their dose of UVB for that treatment.

6. Instruct patients to come out of the light box when the lights have gone out or within 10 seconds of the alarm of the safety (hand-held) timer. Inform patients that the light-box doors are not locked and demonstrate their operation.

7. The list of current medications will be placed in the patient chart and reviewed by the phototherapist. Questions concerning the current medications will be addressed by the attending physician.

8. All patients will be told of the possible complications of UVB phototherapy specifically including

    a. Sunburn reaction
    b. Corneal burn if the eyes are unprotected
    c. Photoallergic dermatitis (including drug reaction)
    d. Freckling of the skin
    e. Aging of the skin
    f. Possible increase in risk of skin cancers

9. Patients will be told that additional unprotected sun exposure should be avoided on the days they receive UVB. Sunblock (SPF 15) should be used on any sun-exposed areas for the remainder of that day.

10. All patients will be given the brochure on UVB phototherapy from the National Psoriasis Foundation.

1. Obtain a signed consent form after the patient has been given the tour of the PTC and basic phototherapy education concerning UVB phototherapy. The patient should be given time for questions.

2. Have the patient undress completely. Male patients should wear an athletic supporter unless otherwise directed or permitted by the attending physician.

3. Eye protection in the form of UV goggles must be worn by all patients when inside the phototherapy unit.

4. The irradiance (mW/cm²) of the UVB light inside the unit should be recorded on a once-a-month basis using the standard method of the manufacturer of the phototherapy unit. Record this irradiance on the phototherapy record sheet or keep an irradiance logbook for the equipment used in patient care.

5. Determine the initial UVB dose (mJ/cm²) according to the patient's skin type as classified by the physician. See Appendix for definitions of skin types.

Skin Type	UVB Dose (mJ/cm²)
Type I	10
Type II	10
Type III	20
Type IV	20
Type V	30
Type VI	30

6. The manual method for calculation of the time (seconds) to set the UVB control panel to deliver the dose from #5 is the following equation: (The measurement of the irradiance can be obtained from the logbook kept on a weekly basis.)

$$\text{Time (seconds)} = \text{Dose (mJ/cm}^2) \div \text{Irradiance (mW/cm}^2)$$

7. The duration of a treatment or total dose of UVB to be delivered can often be calculated by the ultraviolet light unit by following the manufacturer's instructions in the operations manual and inputting the correct information on the control panel prior to the delivery of the treatment.

8. Set the time (or dose) on the control panel of the ultraviolet light unit and on the additional safety timer kept in the light unit or by the technician. In some phototherapy units, the session duration is dependent on the dose measured by an internal photometer, and the time must be estimated by the technician.

9. Verify that the ultraviolet light unit is set on UVB.

10. Turn on the fan and have the patient stand in the center of the ultraviolet light unit with their arms at rest. Double-check that they are wearing UV goggles as eye protection.

11. Instruct the patient to come out of the ultraviolet light box when the lights go out or if they become uncomfortable during the treatment either from burning or stinging of the skin. Inform the patient that the light-box doors are not locked.

12. Start the treatment.

SUBSEQUENT TREATMENTS

13. The frequency of UVB light treatments for the diagnosis of cutaneous T-cell lymphoma is 3 times a week unless otherwise ordered by a physician. If less than 2 times a week has been ordered, then special instructions for the advancement of the dose of UVB light must accompany the request.

14. On subsequent visits, the patient will be asked about redness, light pink color, and tenderness of the skin the previous night, and this information will be put into the phototherapy record.

15. If the skin is red, the phototherapy technician will ask that the patient be seen by the attending physician who will make the decision for adjustment in the UVB treatment. If the skin is a light pink color, the phototherapist should keep the dose the same as the previously delivered treatment dose.

16. Increase the dose (mJ/cm^2) of the UVB light by the amount given down and add it to the previous dose delivered to the patient if the treatment has been within 3 days:

Skin Type	Increase in UVB Dose (mJ/cm^2)
Type I	5
Type II	5
Type III	10
Type IV	10
Type V	20
Type VI	20

17. For subsequent treatments, if the time between treatments has been

4–7 days	Keep the dose the same.
1–2 weeks	Decrease the dose by 50%.
2–3 weeks	Decrease the dose by 75%.
3 or more weeks	Start over.

18. Follow steps 6–12 aforementioned.

19. The dose and frequency of UVB light will be adjusted by the physician according to the response to therapy. The dose of UVB for the diagnosis of cutaneous T-cell lymphoma should not exceed the following guidelines for each skin type:

Skin Type	UVB Dose (mJ/cm²)
Type I	50
Type II	50
Type III	100
Type IV	100
Type V	200
Type VI	200

NARROWBAND ULTRAVIOLET B (NBUVB) PHOTOTHERAPY BY SKIN TYPE

PATIENT INSTRUCTIONS

1. All patients designated for the narrowband ultraviolet B (NBUVB) protocol will have the routine introduction to the PTC facility.

2. All patients designated for the NBUVB protocol will have the basic introduction to phototherapy equipment and safety procedures.

3. Reinforcement of the need for eye protection for all patients and covering of the genital area in males is required.

4. Patients are to stand in the center of the light cabinet with their arms at rest. A step stool may be used for the patients to stand on when recommended by the physician.

5. A hand-held timer will be set by the phototherapy technician for each treatment session. The time will correspond to the estimated time of the treatment session duration, and the timer will either be given to the patients to have with them during the treatment session or be kept by the technician during the treatment. The time will correspond with the amount of time calculated for their dose of NBUVB for that treatment.

6. Instruct patients to come out of the light box when the lights have gone out or within 10 seconds of the alarm of the safety (hand-held) timer. Inform patients that the light-box doors are not locked and demonstrate their operation.

7. The list of current medications will be placed in the patient chart and reviewed by the phototherapist. Questions concerning the current medications will be addressed by the attending physician.

8. All patients will be told of the possible complications of NBUVB phototherapy specifically including

    a. Sunburn reaction
    b. Corneal burn if the eyes are unprotected
    c. Photoallergic dermatitis (including drug reaction)
    d. Freckling of the skin
    e. Aging of the skin
    f. Possible increase in risk of skin cancers

9. Patients will be told that additional unprotected sun exposure should be avoided on the days they receive NBUVB. Sunblock (SPF 15) should be used on any sun-exposed areas for the remainder of that day.

10. All patients will be given the brochure on UVB phototherapy from the National Psoriasis Foundation.

PROTOCOL

1. Obtain a signed consent form after the patient has been given the tour of the PTC and basic phototherapy education concerning NBUVB phototherapy. The patient should be given time for questions.

2. Have the patient undress and expose the areas of CTCL to be treated. Male patients should wear an athletic supporter unless otherwise directed or permitted by the attending physician.

3. Eye protection in the form of UV goggles must be worn by all patients when inside the phototherapy unit.

4. The irradiance (mW/cm^2) of the NBUVB light inside the unit should be recorded on a once-a-week basis using the standard method of the manufacturer of the phototherapy unit. Record this irradiance on the phototherapy record sheet or keep an irradiance logbook for the equipment used in patient care.

5. Determine the initial NBUVB dose (mJ/cm^2) according to the patient's skin type as classified by the physician. See Appendix for definitions of skin types.

Skin Type	NBUVB Dose (mJ/cm²)
Type I	200
Type II	400
Type III	500
Type IV	500
Type V	600
Type VI	600

6. The manual method for calculation of the time (seconds) to set the NBUVB control panel to deliver the dose from #5 is the following equation: (The measurement of the irradiance can be obtained from the logbook kept on a weekly basis.)

$$\text{Time (seconds)} = \text{Dose (mJ/cm}^2) \div \text{Irradiance (mW/cm}^2)$$

7. The duration of a treatment or total dose of NBUVB to be delivered can often be calculated by the ultraviolet light unit by following the manufacturer's instructions in the operations manual and inputting the correct information on the control panel prior to the delivery of the treatment.

8. Set the time (or dose) on the control panel of the ultraviolet light unit and on the additional safety timer kept in the light unit or by the technician. In some phototherapy units, the session duration is dependent on the dose measured by an internal photometer, and the time must be estimated by the technician.

9. Verify that the ultraviolet light unit is set on NBUVB.

10. Turn on the fan and have the patient stand in the center of the ultraviolet light unit with their arms at rest. Double-check that they are wearing UV goggles as eye protection.

11. Instruct the patient to come out of the ultraviolet light box when the lights go out or if they become uncomfortable during the treatment either from burning or stinging of the skin. Inform the patient that the light-box doors are not locked.

12. Start the treatment.

SUBSEQUENT TREATMENTS

13. The frequency of NBUVB light treatments for the diagnosis of CTCL is 3 times a week unless otherwise ordered by a physician. If less than 2 times a week has been ordered by a physician, then special instructions for the advancement of the dose of NBUVB light must accompany the request.

14. On subsequent visits, the patient will be asked about redness, light pink color, and tenderness of the skin the previous night, and this information will be put into the phototherapy record.

15. If the skin is red, the phototherapy technician will ask that the patient be seen by the attending physician who will make the decision for adjustment in the NBUVB treatment. If the skin is a light pink color, the phototherapist should keep the dose the same as the previously delivered treatment dose.

16. Increase the dose (mJ/cm^2) of the NBUVB light by the amount given down and add it to the previous dose delivered to the patient if the treatment has been within 3 days:

    Subsequent treatments—increase by 100 mJ/cm^2

17. Do not exceed 1500 mJ/cm^2 for skin types I–III, and do not exceed 3000 mJ/cm^2 for skin types IV–VI unless otherwise ordered by the physician.

18. For subsequent treatments, if the time between treatments has been

4–7 days	Keep the dose the same.
1–2 weeks	Decrease the dose by 25%.
2–3 weeks	Decrease the dose by 50%.
3 or more weeks	Start over.

19. Follow steps 6–12 aforementioned.

SYSTEMIC PSORALEN PLUS ULTRAVIOLET A TREATMENT

1. All patients designated for the psoralen plus ultraviolet A (PUVA) protocol will have the routine introduction to the PTC facility.

2. All patients designated for the PUVA protocol will have the basic introduction to phototherapy equipment and safety procedures.

3. Reinforcement of the need for eye protection for all patients and covering of the genital area in males is required.

4. Patients receiving systemic PUVA will be instructed to take Oxsoralen Ultra® tablets in the dose prescribed by their physician 1 hour prior to the estimated time of their arrival at the PTC. The treatment will be given between 1 hour 15 minutes and 1 hour 45 minutes after the ingestion of the medication.

5. All patients ingesting Oxsoralen Ultra must wear protective UV blocking glasses when outside, riding in a car, or next to a window from the time they take the medication and for the next 18–24 hours during daylight.

6. Patients are to stand in the center of the light cabinet with their arms at rest. A step stool may be used for the patient to stand on when recommended by the physician.

7. A hand-held timer will be set by the phototherapy technician for each treatment session. The time will correspond to the estimated time of the treatment session duration, and the timer will either be given to the patients to have with them during the treatment session or be kept by the technician during the treatment. The time will correspond with the amount of time calculated for their dose of UVA for that treatment.

8. Instruct patients to come out of the light box when the lights have gone out or within 10 seconds of the alarm of the safety (hand-held) timer. Inform patients that the light-box doors are not locked and demonstrate their operation.

9. The list of current medications will be placed in the patient chart and reviewed by the phototherapist. Questions concerning the current medications will be addressed by the attending physician.

10. All patients will be told of the possible complications of PUVA phototherapy specifically including

    a. Sunburn reaction
    b. Corneal burn if the eyes are unprotected
    c. Cataract formation if the eyes are unprotected
    d. Photoallergic dermatitis (including drug reaction)

  e. Freckling of the skin
  f. Aging of the skin
  g. Increase in risk of skin cancers including melanoma

11. Patients will be told that additional unprotected sun exposure should be avoided on the days they receive PUVA. Wide-spectrum sunblock (UVA/B) should be used on any sun-exposed areas for the remainder of that day.

12. All patients will be given the brochure on PUVA phototherapy from the National Psoriasis Foundation.

PROTOCOL

1. The diagnosis of T-cell lymphoma of the skin or mycosis fungoides must be documented and on the chart at the time of referral to the PTC.

2. Obtain a signed consent form after the patient has been given the tour of the PTC and basic phototherapy education concerning PUVA phototherapy. The patient should be given time for questions.

3. Oxsoralen Ultra (8-methoxypsoralen) is to be ingested by the patient at least 1 hour prior to arrival at the PTC. Treatments may be given anytime between 1 hour 15 minutes and 1 hour 45 minutes after ingestion.

4. Dosage of the Oxsoralen Ultra tablets is dependent on the orders of the attending physician and will vary from patient to patient. The standard dosage is 0.5–0.6 mg/kg.

5. Ask the patient at what time they ingested their medication and how many pills they ingested.

6. Have the patient undress so that all affected areas that are to be treated are exposed to the UV light. Male patients should wear an athletic supporter unless otherwise directed or permitted by the attending physician.

7. Eye protection in the form of UV goggles must be worn by all patients when inside the phototherapy unit. The only exception to this rule will be by physician orders.

8. The irradiance (mW/cm^2) of the UVA light inside the unit should be recorded on a once-a-month basis using the standard method of the manufacturer of the phototherapy unit. Record this irradiance on the phototherapy record sheet or keep an irradiance logbook for the equipment used in patient care.

9. Determine the initial PUVA dose (J/cm^2) according to the patient's skin type as classified by the physician. See Appendix for definitions of skin types.

Skin Type	Initial UVA Dose (J/cm^2)
Type I	1
Type II	1
Type III	1
Type IV	2
Type V	2
Type VI	2

10. The manual method for calculation of the time (seconds) to set the UVA control panel to deliver the dose from #9 is the following equation: (The measurement of the irradiance can be obtained from the logbook kept on a weekly basis.)

$$\text{Time (seconds)} = \text{Dose } (mJ/cm^2) \div \text{Irradiance } (mW/cm^2)$$

11. The duration of a treatment or total dose of UVA to be delivered can often be calculated by the ultraviolet light unit by following the manufacturer's instructions in the operations manual and inputting the correct information on the control panel prior to the delivery of the treatment.

12. Set the time (or dose) on the control panel of the ultraviolet light unit and on the additional safety timer kept in the light unit or by the technician. In some phototherapy units, the session duration is dependent on the dose measured by an internal photometer, and the time must be estimated by the technician.

13. Verify that the ultraviolet light unit is set on UVA.

14. Turn on the fan and have the patient stand in the center of the ultraviolet light unit with arms at rest. Double-check that they are wearing UV goggles as eye protection.

15. Instruct the patient to come out of the ultraviolet light box when the lights go out or if they become uncomfortable during the treatment either from burning or stinging of the skin. Inform the patient that the light-box doors are not locked.

16. Start the treatment.

17. Some patients may receive localized ultraviolet light therapy to the legs or trunk as ordered by the physician.

SUBSEQUENT TREATMENTS

18. The frequency of PUVA treatments for the diagnosis of cutaneous T-cell lymphoma is 2–3 times a week unless otherwise ordered by a physician. If less than 2 times a week has been ordered, then special instructions for the advancement of the dose of UVA light must accompany the request.

19. On subsequent visits, the patient will be asked about redness, light pink color, and tenderness of the skin the previous night, and this information will be put into the phototherapy record. The patient will also be asked at what time they took the Oxsoralen Ultra tablets.

20. If the skin is red, the phototherapist will ask that the patient be seen by the attending physician who will make the decision for adjustment in the treatment for that day. If the skin is a light pink color, the phototherapist should keep the dose the same as the previously delivered treatment dose.

21. Increase the dose (J/cm^2) of the UVA light by 1.0 J/cm^2 each treatment up to a dose of 8 J/cm^2 for skin types I–III, and 12 J/cm^2 for skin types IV–VI, then hold that dose unless ordered by the physician.

22. For subsequent treatments, if the time between treatments has been

1 week	Keep the dose the same.
2 weeks	Decrease the dose by 25%.
3 weeks	Decrease the dose by 50%.
4 weeks	Start over.

23. Further increases in the dose of UVA light will be by the direction of the physician.

24. Follow steps 3–16 aforementioned.

25. An ophthalmology examination should be performed prior to and every 6 months during therapy.

26. Laboratory monitoring may be done at baseline and every 6 months as needed.

Scleroderma and Other Sclerosing Disorders

BROAD BAND ULTRAVIOLET A PHOTOTHERAPY BY FIXED DOSE

1. All patients designated for the ultraviolet A (UVA) will have the routine introduction to the Phototherapy Treatment Center (PTC) facility.

2. All patients designated for the broad band UVA protocol will have the basic introduction to phototherapy equipment and safety procedures.

3. Reinforcement of the need for eye protection and covering of the genital area in males is required.

4. All patients with the diagnosis of psoriasis will be told to apply mineral oil to the involved areas of the skin prior to the delivery of UVA.

5. Patients are to stand in the center of the light cabinet with their arms at rest. A step stool may be used for the patients to stand on when recommended by the physician.

6. A hand-held timer will be set by the phototherapy technician for each treatment session. The time will correspond to the estimated time of the treatment session duration, and the timer will either be given to the patient to have with them during the treatment session or be kept by the technician during the treatment. The time will correspond with the amount of time calculated for their dose of UVA for that treatment.

7. Instruct patients to come out of the light box when the lights have gone out or within 10 seconds of the alarm of the safety (hand-held) timer. Inform patients that the light-box doors are not locked and demonstrate their operation.

8. The list of current medications will be placed in the patient chart and reviewed by the phototherapist. Questions concerning the current medications will be addressed by the attending physician.

9. All patients will be told of the possible complications of UVA phototherapy specifically including

    a. Sunburn reaction
    b. Corneal burn if the eyes are unprotected
    c. Photoallergic dermatitis (including drug reaction)
    d. Freckling of the skin
    e. Aging of the skin
    f. Possible increase in risk of skin cancers

10. Patients will be told that additional unprotected sun exposure should be avoided on the days they receive UVA. Broad-spectrum sunblock (SPF 15) should be used on any sun-exposed areas for the remainder of that day.

11. All patients will be given the brochure on UV phototherapy from the National Psoriasis Foundation.

1. Obtain a signed consent form after the patient has been given the tour of the PTC and basic phototherapy education concerning UVA phototherapy. The patient should be given time for questions.

2. Have the patient undress completely and apply mineral oil to areas of psoriasis prior to the treatment. Male patients should wear an athletic supporter unless otherwise directed or permitted by the attending physician.

3. Eye protection in the form of UV goggles must be worn by all patients when inside the phototherapy unit.

4. The irradiance (mW/cm^2) of the UVA light inside the unit should be recorded on a once-a-month basis using the standard method of the manufacturer of the phototherapy unit. Record this irradiance on the phototherapy record sheet or keep an irradiance logbook for the equipment used in patient care.

5. The initial UVA dose (J/cm^2) will be 20 J/cm^2.

6. The manual method for calculation of the time (seconds) to set the UVA control panel to deliver the dose is the following equation: (The measurement of the irradiance can be obtained from the logbook kept on a weekly basis.)

$$\text{Time (seconds)} = \text{Dose (20 J/cm}^2) \div \text{Irradiance (W/cm}^2)$$

7. The duration of a treatment or total dose of UVA to be delivered can often be calculated by the ultraviolet light unit by following the manufacturer's instructions in the operations manual and inputting the correct information on the control panel prior to the delivery of the treatment.

8. Set the time (or dose) on the control panel of the ultraviolet light unit and on the additional safety timer kept in the light unit or by the technician. In some phototherapy units, the session duration is dependent on the dose measured by an internal photometer, and the time must be estimated by the technician.

9. Verify that the ultraviolet light unit is set on UVA.

10. Turn on the fan and have the patient stand in the center of the ultraviolet light unit with their arms at rest. Double-check that they are wearing goggles as eye protection.

11. Instruct the patient to come out of the ultraviolet light box when the lights go out or if they become uncomfortable during the treatment either from burning or stinging of the skin. Inform the patient that the light-box doors are not locked.

12. Start the treatment.

SUBSEQUENT TREATMENTS

13. The frequency of UVA for the diagnosis of scleroderma/morphea is 3 times a week unless otherwise ordered by a physician.

14. On subsequent visits, the patient will be asked about redness, light pink color, and tenderness of the skin the previous night, and this information will be put into the phototherapy record.

15. If the skin is a light pink color, the phototherapist should keep the dose the same as the previously delivered treatment dose.

16. If the skin is red, the phototherapy technician will ask that the patient be seen by the attending physician who will make the decision for adjustment in the UVB treatment.

ULTRAVIOLET A1 (UVA1) PHOTOTHERAPY BY FIXED DOSE

PATIENT INSTRUCTIONS

1. All patients designated for the UVA1 will have the routine introduction to the PTC facility.

2. All patients designated for the UVA1 protocol will have the basic introduction to phototherapy equipment and safety procedures.

3. Reinforcement of the need for eye protection and covering of the genital area in males is required.

4. All patients with the diagnosis of psoriasis will be told to apply mineral oil to the involved areas of the skin prior to the delivery of UVA1.

5. Patients are to lie in the light cabinet with arms at rest.

6. A hand-held timer will be set by the phototherapy technician for each treatment session. The time will correspond to the estimated time of the treatment session duration, and the timer will either be given to the patient to have with them during the treatment session or be kept by the technician during the treatment. The time will correspond with the amount of time calculated for their dose of UVA1 for that treatment.

7. Instruct patients to come out of the light unit when the lights have gone out or within 10 seconds of the alarm of the safety (hand-held) timer.

8. The list of current medications will be placed in the patient chart and reviewed by the phototherapist. Questions concerning the current medications will be addressed by the attending physician.

9. All patients will be told of the possible complications of UVA1 phototherapy specifically including

   a. Sunburn reaction
   b. Corneal burn if the eyes are unprotected
   c. Photoallergic dermatitis (including drug reaction)
   d. Freckling of the skin
   e. Aging of the skin
   f. Possible increase in risk of skin cancers

10. Patients will be told that additional unprotected sun exposure should be avoided on the days they receive UVA. Broad-spectrum sunblock (SPF 15) should be used on any sun-exposed areas for the remainder of that day.

11. All patients will be given the brochure on UV phototherapy from the National Psoriasis Foundation.

PROTOCOL

1. Obtain a signed consent form after the patient has been given the tour of the PTC and basic phototherapy education concerning UVA phototherapy. The patient should be given time for questions.

2. Have the patient undress completely and apply mineral oil to areas of psoriasis prior to the treatment. Male patients should wear an athletic supporter unless otherwise directed or permitted by the attending physician.

3. Eye protection in the form of UV goggles must be worn by all patients when inside the phototherapy unit.

4. The irradiance (mW/cm^2) of the UVA light inside the unit should be recorded on a once-a-month basis using the standard method of the manufacturer of the phototherapy unit. Record this irradiance on the phototherapy record sheet or keep an irradiance logbook for the equipment used in patient care.

5. The initial UVA dose (J/cm^2) will be determined as follows:

UVA1 Dosing Recommendations

Indications	UVA1 Dosage
Atopic dermatitis or cutaneous T-cell lymphoma	Medium-dose 60 J/cm^2 3–5 times weekly for 3–6 weeks
Localized scleroderma	Medium-dose 60 J/cm^2 3–5 times weekly for 40 sessions
Lichen sclerosus	Medium-dose 50 J/cm^2 5 times per week for 40 sessions
Systemic lupus erythematosus	Low-dose 10 J/cm^2 5 times per week for 3 weeks
Subacute prurigo	Medium-dose 50 J/cm^2 5 times per week for 4 weeks
Urticaria pigmentosa	Medium-dose 60 J/cm^2 5 times weekly for 3 weeks
Pityriasis rosea	Medium-dose 30 J/cm^2 3 times weekly for 3 weeks

Source: Adapted from Gambichler, T. et al., *Clin. Dermatol.*, 31, 438, 2013.

6. The manual method for calculation of the time (seconds) to set the UVA control panel to deliver the dose is the following equation: (The measurement of the irradiance can be obtained from the logbook kept on a weekly basis.)

$$\text{Time (seconds)} = \text{Dose } (J/cm^2) \div \text{Irradiance } (W/cm^2)$$

7. The duration of a treatment or total dose of UVA1 to be delivered can often be calculated by the ultraviolet light unit by following the manufacturer's instructions in the operations manual and inputting the correct information on the control panel prior to the delivery of the treatment.

8. Set the time (or dose) on the control panel of the ultraviolet light unit and on the additional safety timer kept in the light unit or by the technician. In some phototherapy units, the session duration is dependent on the dose

measured by an internal photometer, and the time must be estimated by the technician.

9. Verify that the ultraviolet light unit is set on UVA.

10. Turn on the fan and have the patient lie in the center of the ultraviolet light unit with their arms at rest. Double-check that they are wearing goggles as eye protection.

11. Instruct the patient to come out of the ultraviolet light unit when the lights go out or if they become uncomfortable during the treatment either from burning or stinging of the skin. Inform the patient that the light-box doors are not locked.

12. Start the treatment.

SUBSEQUENT TREATMENTS

13. The frequency of UVA1 is 3–5 times a week as ordered by a physician (see recommendation table).

14. On subsequent visits, the patient will be asked about redness, light pink color, and tenderness of the skin the previous night, and this information will be put into the phototherapy record.

15. If the skin is a light pink color, the phototherapist should keep the dose the same as the previously delivered treatment dose.

16. If the skin is red, the phototherapy technician will ask that the patient be seen by the attending physician who will make the decision for adjustment in the UVB treatment.

REFERENCE
Gambichler T et al. Treatment regimens, protocols, dosage, and indications for UVA1 phototherapy: Facts and controversies. *Clin. Dermatol.*, 31, 438–454, 2013.

Other Phototherapy-Responsive Dermatologic Diseases That May Be Treated with Selected Protocols

UVB PROTOCOL FOR ATOPIC DERMATITIS (P. 91)
This can also be used for

> Eosinophilic folliculitis
> Pityriasis rosea

NARROWBAND UVB PROTOCOL FOR CTCL (P. 128)
This can also be used for

> Eosinophilic folliculitis
> Graft vs. host disease
> Granuloma annulare
> Lichen planus
> Parapsoriasis
> > Small plaque type
> > Large plaque type
> Polymorphous light eruption
> Pityriasis rosea

PUVA PROTOCOL FOR CTCL (P. 131)
This can also be used for

Graft vs. host disease
Granuloma annulare
Lichen planus
Parapsoriasis
    Small plaque type
    Large plaque type
Polymorphous light eruption
Urticaria pigmentosa
Scleroderma and morphea

Patient Consent Forms

ULTRAVIOLET B PHOTOTHERAPY CONSENT

Ultraviolet B (UVB) light is the most common form of phototherapy used to treat various skin diseases, including psoriasis, eczema, and itching. You will be exposed to this high-energy UV light for a varying length of time. This treatment is NOT A CURE but can effectively control or improve your disease. Patients have used this treatment successfully for many years and often are able to maintain clearance of improved skin over extended periods of time.

Each condition and patient will vary in the number of treatments needed per week and the time it will take to reach clearing. Most patients initially require three to five treatments each week to clear their lesions. Typically, treatments start with only a few seconds of light exposure and increase gradually as determined by the staff. It may take 15–25 treatments or longer to improve your disease. Not all patients will clear completely. Many patients go into remission and may then stop treatments.

The expected benefits of phototherapy are as follows:

1. Improvement of existing lesions.

2. Reduction of new lesions.

3. Remission—in many cases phototherapy has resulted in a near-total clearing of the disease process. The duration of this remission varies with each patient. Maintenance therapy may be required.

Risks and side effects of phototherapy are as follows:

4. The most common side effect of this therapy is UVB-induced sunburn. This may occur at any time during therapy. Certain drugs may also cause you to get sunburn. Please let your doctor/nurse know of any medications you are taking, or any that you begin while undergoing therapy.

5. It is possible with any form of UV light that an increased incidence of skin cancer may occur later in some patients, usually only with many UV light treatments.

6. UV treatments may cause dryness and itching.

7. UV treatments age the skin over time and may increase freckles and pigmentation of the skin.

8. UV rays may damage the eyes and increase your risk of cataracts. This is preventable with protective eye goggles worn during treatment. These will be given to you and are required for treatment.

9. UV light may cause a flare of fever blisters and mouth sores in susceptible people.

10. Long-term UV exposure to the unprotected genital area in men may cause an increase in genital cancer. Therefore, all men will wear an athletic supporter while in the light box.

11. UV light may cause exacerbation of other medical conditions, such as lupus erythematosus, which have sensitivity to UV wavelength.

Should you have any questions concerning any aspect of your treatment, please call the Phototherapy Treatment Center.

I have fully explained to the patient, _____ the nature, purpose, and expected benefits of phototherapy, as well as the risks. I have also explained the alternative treatments and their potential risk. I will answer any questions regarding the procedure.

Physician/Physician Assistant/Nurse Practitioner/_____ Date _____
Phototherapy Technician_____

I have fully read and understood the above information regarding UVB therapy. I also understand that no one completely knows the long-term effects of phototherapy. I realize that these treatments do not cure my skin disorder and that I may need maintenance therapy. I authorize my doctor (above) to prescribe light therapy.

This authorization extends to his associates, including other physicians and assistants selected by him/her, to carry out phototherapy. I understand that I am free to withdraw my consent and stop treatment at any time.

Patient Signature (or Legal Guardian)_____

Witness Signature_____ Date _____

NARROWBAND ULTRAVIOLET B (NBUVB) PHOTOTHERAPY CONSENT

UVB (ultraviolet B light) is the most common form of phototherapy and is used to treat various skin diseases, including psoriasis, eczema, and itching. You will be exposed to this high-energy UV light for a varying length of time. This treatment is NOT A CURE but can effectively control or improve your disease. Patients have used this treatment successfully for many years and often are able to maintain clearance of improved skin over extended periods of time.

Each condition and patient will vary in the number of treatments needed per week and the time it will take to reach clearing. Most patients initially require three to five treatments each week to clear their lesions. Typically, treatments start with only a few seconds of light exposure and increase gradually as determined by the staff. It may take 15–25 treatments or longer to improve your disease. Not all patients will clear completely. Many patients go into remission and may then stop treatments.

The expected benefits of phototherapy are as follows:

1. Improvement of existing lesions.

2. Reduction of new lesions.

3. Remission—in many cases phototherapy has resulted in a near-total clearing of the disease process. The duration of this remission varies with each patient. Maintenance therapy may be required.

Risks and side effects of phototherapy are as follows:

1. The most common side effect of this therapy is UVB-induced sunburn. This may occur at any time during therapy. Certain drugs may also cause you to get sunburn. Please let your doctor/nurse know of any medications you are taking, or any that you begin while undergoing therapy.

2. It is possible with any form of UV light that an increased incidence of skin cancer may occur later in some patients, usually only with many UV light treatments.

3. UV treatments may cause dryness and itching.

4. UV treatments age the skin over time and may increase freckles and pigmentation of the skin.

5. UV rays may damage the eyes and increase your risk of cataracts. This is preventable with protective eye goggles worn during treatment. These will be given to you and are required for treatment.

6. UV light may cause a flare of fever blisters and mouth sores in susceptible people.

7. Long-term UV exposure to the unprotected genital area in men may cause an increase in genital cancer. Therefore, all men will wear an athletic supporter while in the light box.

8. UV light may cause exacerbation of other medical conditions, such as lupus erythematosus, which have sensitivity to UV wavelength.

Should you have any questions concerning any aspect of your treatment, please call the Phototherapy Treatment Center.

I have fully explained to the patient, _____,
the nature, purpose, and expected benefits of phototherapy, as well as the risks. I have also explained the alternative treatments and their potential risk. I will answer any questions regarding the procedure.

Physician/Physician Assistant/Nurse Practitioner/_____ Date _____
Phototherapy Technician_____

I have fully read and understood the above information regarding UVB therapy. I also understand that no one completely knows the long-term effects of phototherapy. I realize that these treatments do not cure my skin disorder and that I may need maintenance therapy. I authorize my doctor (above) to prescribe light therapy.

This authorization extends to his associates, including other physicians and assistants selected by him/her, to carry out phototherapy. I understand that I am free to withdraw my consent and stop treatment at any time.

Patient Signature (or Legal Guardian)_____

Witness Signature_____ Date _____

PSORALEN PLUS ULTRAVIOLET A (PUVA) CONSENT

PUVA therapy is a combined drug and ultraviolet light program. You will take a psoralen (Oxsoralen Ultra) medication before you get into a special ultraviolet A (UVA) light box. PUVA was first developed in 1974 and has been used to treat a variety of skin disorders including psoriasis, vitiligo, mycosis fungoides, and various other skin conditions. This treatment is NOT A CURE but may effectively control or improve your disease.

The psoralen medication may be taken by pill form (systemic PUVA) or by soaking in a topical solution (bath PUVA). The medication makes the skin more sensitive to the UVA light, which makes the light work more effectively.

Each condition and patient will vary in the number of treatments needed. Initially, the treatment will start with only a few minutes of light exposure, and then may gradually increase to approximately 20 minutes of exposure depending on patient tolerance and skin condition being treated. The average patient requires two to three treatments per week. Most psoriasis and eczema patients require 15–20 treatments to improve the disease. Mycosis fungoides and vitiligo often need more treatments. After clearing, some patients continue with maintenance treatments every 2–4 weeks for many months.

The expected benefits of PUVA phototherapy are as follows:

1. Improvement of existing lesions.

2. Reduction of new lesions.

3. Remission—in many cases phototherapy has resulted in a near-total clearing of the disease process. The duration of remission varies with each patient. Maintenance therapy may be required.

Risks and side effects of PUVA phototherapy are as follows:

1. Occasional nausea and stomach upset when taking pills for systemic PUVA. This can be corrected by taking the pills with food.

2. An exaggerated sunburn. The drug stays in the skin for up to 24 hours after it has been taken.

   Avoid sun exposure after the treatment. Protect yourself with clothing and sunscreen. Sunburn reactions from psoralen can be life-threatening, so do not expose yourself to sunlight or tanning beds after taking the medications. It may take 1–2 days for this sunburn to first show up and may last for several days. Certain drugs may also increase light sensitivity. Please let your doctor/nurse know of any medications you are taking.

3. It is possible with any form of UV light that an increased incidence of skin cancer (including melanoma) may occur later in some patients, usually only with many UV light treatments.

4. UV treatments may cause dryness and itching.

5.   UV treatments age the skin over time and may increase freckles and pigmentation of the skin.

6.   UV rays may damage the eyes and increase your risk of cataracts. This is preventable with protective eye goggles worn during treatment. Systemic PUVA patients must also wear UV-protective eye goggles for up to 24 hours after treatment since the pills make your eyes more sensitive to light.

7.   UV light may cause a flare of fever blisters and mouth ulcers in susceptible people.

8.   Long-term UV exposure to the unprotected genital area in men may cause an increase in genital cancer. Therefore, all men will wear an athletic supporter while in the light box.

9.   UV light may cause exacerbation of other medical conditions, such as lupus erythematosus, which have sensitivity to UV wavelength.

Should you have questions concerning any aspect of your treatment, please call the Phototherapy Treatment Center.

I have fully explained to the patient,_____,
the nature, purpose, and expected benefits of phototherapy, as well as the risks. I have also explained the alternative treatments and their potential risk. I will answer any questions regarding the procedure.

Physician/Physician Assistant/Nurse Practitioner/_____ Date _____
Phototherapy Technician_____

I have fully read and understood the above information regarding PUVA therapy. I also understand that no one completely knows the long-term effects of phototherapy. I realize that these treatments do not cure my skin disorder and that I may need maintenance therapy. I authorize my doctor (above) to prescribe light therapy.

This authorization extends to his associates, including other physicians and assistants selected by him/her, to carry out phototherapy. I understand that I am free to withdraw my consent and stop treatment at any time.

_____   _____   _____

Patient Signature   Witness Signature   Date
(or Legal Guardian)

SCALP TREATMENTS CONSENT

I understand I will undergo specialized treatments for my scalp disease. Medication will be applied to my scalp and then washed out. This treatment is not a cure but may improve my disease.

The procedure for the scalp treatment will include the following:

1. P&S Liquid will be applied onto my scalp to coat and protect my scalp.

2. Anthralin will be applied to my scalp if needed.

3. I will cover my scalp with a plastic cover and wait 30 minutes. I will have a towel around my neck and a washcloth to catch any of the medication that drips. I will try not to let any of the medication drip into my mouth or eyes.

4. My scalp will then be rinsed with detergent.

5. My scalp will then be rinsed in the scalp machine with a combination of warm water and shampoo. The machine will wash my scalp for 20 minutes.

I will notify my physician and his staff if I am aware of any sensitivity to any of the above ingredients. The expected benefits of scalp treatments include

1. Improvement of existing lesions

2. Reduction of new lesions

Some of the risks and side effects of the scalp treatments include the following:

1. Possible irritation (itching, burning) to my scalp.

2. Possible irritation to my eyes if the medication drips into them. This may include burning, tearing, pain, and visual changes. I will notify my physician at once should I have any of these symptoms. My physician may arrange for me to be seen by an ophthalmologist if necessary.

If I have any questions concerning my treatment, I may call the Phototherapy Treatment Center.

I have fully read and understood the above information concerning scalp treatments.

I realize that these treatments may not cure my skin disorder. I have been advised of the most frequent risks and consequences of scalp treatments and of the alternative treatments available to me. Even with this information I elect to proceed with scalp treatments.

I authorize my doctor to prescribe scalp treatments. This authorization extends to his associates, including other physicians and assistants selected by him/her to carry out the treatments. I understand I am free to withdraw my consent and stop treatment at any time.

_____   _____

Patient Signature (or Legal Guardian)   Date

_____   _____

Witness Signature   Date

HOME ULTRAVIOLET THERAPY CONSENT

I understand that I am using ultraviolet (UV) type B therapy for my skin disease. I understand that I must take the following precautions:

1. I will wear the specified UV-protective goggles during treatment. Failure to wear protective goggles may result in severe burns or long-term injury to eyes.

2. I will stand no closer than 6–8 in. from the light source and stand at the same distance for each treatment. I will not touch the UV bulbs when they are turned on.

3. I will set the machine timer carefully as recommended by the manufacturer to avoid burning my skin.

4. I will be seen by my dermatologist every 6 months for routine skin examination. This is to ensure that the UV light is not causing damage to my skin.

5. If I cannot see my dermatologist at these times, I must STOP using the UV treatment.

6. I understand that UV light boxes are made by different companies and may have different operating instructions. I will comply with the manufacturer's instructions provided with my light box. My dermatologist may also advise me on refining my treatment plan.

7. I will not wear any cosmetics or fragrances during UV light treatments.

8. I agree to notify my dermatologist before I take any new medications, as some medications may increase sensitivity to UV light.

9. I understand that home UV treatments may have side effects such as allergic reactions, burning of the skin, a possible increased risk of skin cancer, increased aging of the skin, including wrinkles, freckles, loss of skin tone, and color changes, and other less common side effects.

10. I have been advised of the most frequent risks and consequences of UV light treatment and of the alternative treatments available to me. Even with this information I elect to proceed with home UV light therapy.

_____   _____

Patient's Signature   Date

Patient Educational Handouts

ULTRAVIOLET B PHOTOTHERAPY PATIENT INFORMATION

Ultraviolet B (UVB) phototherapy involves standing in a light box, a closed-in cubicle that is lined with ultraviolet lights. You will not be locked into the light cabinet. You may open the doors and exit the booth at any time during the treatment. In the beginning, treatment sessions may last around 20 seconds. Treatment times slowly increase, depending on patient tolerance and skin disease being treated.

Please follow the guidelines given down to assure a smooth and productive treatment experience:

1. Males are required to wear an athletic supporter while in the light box. Females will undress completely for their treatment unless otherwise instructed by their physician.

2. You will be given a pair of protective eye goggles. You are required to wear them during the light exposure.

3. While you are in the light cabinet, stand in the middle at a normal stance. The lights are on all the panels plus reflector sheets, which dispense the light rays for uniform exposure.

4. For psoriasis patients, apply mineral oil to your skin prior to exposure to the light. This will decrease dryness and enhance the effectiveness of the light.

5. Please notify the staff of any redness and/or tenderness you have during your treatment. At home, cool compresses and aspirin are helpful for mild sunburn reactions.

6. Notify the staff if you begin any new medications during your treatment, as certain medications affect your sensitivity to UV light.

7. All patients should use moisturizers frequently.

8. Avoid additional sunlight on the day of treatment to prevent burning.

9. Children undergoing UVB must be accompanied to the Phototherapy Treatment Center (PTC) by a parent.

10. Timers are provided in the light boxes for your use so that you will be fully aware of the amount of time you receive light. The light boxes also have timers, but backup timers promote safety.

SYSTEMIC PUVA PATIENT INFORMATION

1. You will take a certain number (prescribed by your physician) of psoralen (Oxsoralen Ultra) tablets. Take them between 1 and 1½ hours before your treatment. Take the pills with food (bread, crackers, cereal, and sandwich) or milk. Avoid greasy, spicy foods, when you take your pills. *Be consistent with what foods or liquids are taken with the psoralen drug.*

2. The psoralen makes your skin and eyes more sensitive to light. Wear sunscreen, protective clothing, and protective glasses (we will give these to you) from the time you take your medicine for the next 24 hours. You should wear these glasses even inside your car, and inside a building if it has glass windows. Since the lenses of your eyes are more sensitive to the ultraviolet light, the possibility of cataract formation increases. Wearing your protective sunglasses will minimize the risk. PLEASE SCHEDULE AN APPOINTMENT WITH AN *OPHTHALMOLOGIST* FOR A BASELINE EXAM. Our receptionist can help schedule an appointment with an ophthalmologist.

3. Avoid getting extra sunlight or using a tanning bed while undergoing PUVA.

4. You will stand in a closed cubicle that emits UVA light. The door is *not* locked. You may leave the unit at anytime. A backup timer will be provided to you for safety purposes. Stand in the middle of the light box at a normal stance.

5. You will be given a pair of protective goggles to wear during your light treatment. Bring these with you to each treatment.

6. Males are required to wear an athletic supporter. Females will undress completely unless otherwise directed by their doctor.

7. Notify your doctor if you are pregnant, have cataracts, or a history of skin cancer.

8. You may experience skin burning while taking this treatment. Please notify the PTC of any redness and tenderness at your next visit. Notify the Center immediately if severe burning occurs.

9. Be advised that potential, long-term risks of PUVA therapy are premature skin aging, development of cataracts, and skin cancers including melanomas.

10. Store your psoralen medication away from heat and light. Keep out of reach of children. Do not share your medication with others.

11. Should you have any questions concerning your treatment, please call the PTC.

TOPICAL BATH/PAINT PUVA PATIENT INFORMATION

Bath PUVA therapy involves soaking of the hands/feet in a photosensitizing solution followed by administration of ultraviolet A light (P for the psoralen soak and UVA for the ultraviolet A light). In paint PUVA, medication is applied to the affected areas with a Q-tip, then you are exposed to the UVA light. These therapies are used to treat various skin disorders of the hands, feet, face, or body such as psoriasis, atopic dermatitis, vitiligo, and eczema. Treatments are generally taken 2–3 times a week and are usually not given on consecutive days. Please read the following information so that you will have a better understanding of your therapy:

1. For bath PUVA, you will soak your hands/feet in a warm solution containing the liquid psoralen drug. You will soak for 15 minutes. Please notify the nurse of any sores, cuts, or drainage on your hands or feet. After soaking, dry your hands and feet well. Sunscreen will be applied to your wrists and back of hand to protect these areas from the ultraviolet rays.

2. For paint PUVA, the phototherapists will apply the psoralen medication to the affected areas. You will wait 30 minutes for the medication to soak in. To avoid getting the psoralen medication on your hands, do not touch the treated areas.

3. You will be given protective glasses to wear during the light therapy. These will shield your eyes from the ultraviolet rays. For added protection, wear the glasses for 1 hour after the treatment.

4. After the light treatment, wash and dry the treated area thoroughly and apply the sunscreen provided. Avoid excessive sun exposure to the treated area for the remainder of the day, and keep sunscreen on for the next 24 hours.

5. Your initial time for light exposure will be brief. We will increase your exposure to the UVA rays gradually.

6. Occasionally, some patients experience a skin burning while undergoing this treatment. Severe burns with blistering can occur. Please notify the Phototherapy center if this should occur.

7. Should you have any questions or concerns, call the PTC.

GOECKERMAN REGIMEN PATIENT INFORMATION

The Goeckerman program, as it is used today to clear psoriasis, is one of the most effective treatment programs available, has few side effects, and is cost-effective in a treatment center setting. In the past, the Goeckerman program was administered mainly in a hospital.

Treatments are given daily (Monday–Friday), and they last approximately 6–8 hours. Following this daily regimen is most important for the treatments to be successful. It takes an average of 20–25 treatments to clear the skin. The average amount of time people remain clear (remission period) after completing treatments is an average of 6–12 months.

We begin treatments between 8:30 and 9:00 a.m. We recommend that valuables, especially jewelry, be left at home as we cannot assume responsibility for lost items.

First, you will receive light treatment. Afterward, we will apply a coal tar mixture to your body. You will then be wrapped in a plastic dressing. A scrub suit will be provided for you to wear while wrapped in the tar. You must stay within the hospital while the tar is on your body. You will need an old pair of slippers or thongs to wear in the Center. You will have the tar on your skin for around 6 hours. (Additional topical medications may be added in the afternoon if indicated.) After this full day of topical treatment, you will be ready to shower. Make sure the tar is completely washed off. We provide soap and shampoo. Please bring your own moisturizer. It is important to keep your skin well-lubricated.

This treatment is intensive, but hopefully you will find that our qualified, understanding staff and new facilities help the time in treatment to pass more quickly. The PTC is equipped with a refrigerator and microwave for your use. The PTC also has a lounge equipped with a telephone, television, and VCR. Various movies for entertainment and education are available for your viewing while in treatment. If you should need a place to stay in the area while in treatment, the Medical Center has a hotel nearby that offers a free shuttle service.

We can also assist you with making arrangements to stay in an inexpensive boarding home or hotel with suitable amenities. It is advisable that you bring some old sheets to sleep in as you may need to apply tar at bed time as well.

We welcome you to the PTC! You are encouraged to communicate any concerns, questions, or recommendations to our staff. We hope that you will have a pleasant and successful experience at our Center.

MODIFIED INGRAM PATIENT INFORMATION

The Modified Ingram program consists of ultraviolet A (UVA) or B (UVB) phototherapy and the topical application of Anthralin. Anthralin is a synthetic substance made from anthracene, a coal tar derivative, and has been used in the treatment of psoriasis since the nineteenth century. Anthralin may temporarily stain skin during treatment. It can permanently stain clothes.

Treatments are given daily (Monday–Friday) and last approximately 2–4 hours. Following this daily regimen is most important for the treatments to be successful. It takes an average of 20–25 treatments to clear the skin.

We begin treatments between 8 a.m. and 1 p.m. We recommend that valuables, especially jewelry, be left at home as we can assume no responsibility for lost items. First, you will receive your UVB or UVA light treatment. Afterward, we will apply an Anthralin paste to your psoriasis. Petroleum jelly will be applied to the surrounding normal skin to prevent irritation from the Anthralin. Talc powder is then applied to prevent the Anthralin from smearing. You are then wrapped in a plastic dressing. A scrub suit will be provided for you to wear while wrapped in the Anthralin. You must stay within the hospital while the Anthralin is on your body. You will need an old pair of slippers or thongs to wear while in the Center.

After leaving the Anthralin on at least 2 hours, you will be ready to shower. Make sure the Anthralin is completely washed off. We provide soap and shampoo. Please bring your own moisturizer. It is important to keep your skin well-lubricated.

This treatment is intensive, but hopefully you will find that our qualified staff and treatment facilities help the time in treatment pass more quickly. The PTC is equipped with a refrigerator, microwave, telephone, TV, and VCR. Various movies for entertainment and education are available for your viewing while in treatment.

We welcome you to the PTC. You are encouraged to communicate any concerns, questions, or recommendations to our staff. We hope you will have a pleasant and successful experience at our Center.

Treatment Management Forms

PHYSICIAN'S ORDERS

NAME: _____

DIAGNOSIS: PSORIASIS   PLEVA   CTCL

                     ATOPIC DERMATITIS   HAND ECZEMA   ALOPECIA

                     PRURITUS   PITYRIASIS ROSEA   VITILIGO

                     NEURODERMATITIS

                     OTHER:_____

DATE:_____

DOCTOR'S ORDERS:

Type of Treatment	Frequency of Treatment			Special Instructions
	Per Protocol	Times/Week	Times/Month	
UVB				
NBUVB				
PUVA				
Goeckerman				
Modified Ingram				
UVA/UVB (combined)				
Hand/foot (UVA or UVB)				
Scalp treatment				
Hydrosound				
Iontophoresis				
Other				

Current medications: _____

_____

_____

Skin type (for ultraviolet light treatments):   I   II   III   IV   V   VI

Consent obtained (required for any ultraviolet light treatment):   YES   NO

Ophthalmologic examination (for PUVA treatments):   YES   NO

Comments :

M.D./P.A./R.N.P. signature: _____

TREATMENT RECORD

Pt. name _____   Diagnosis _____

Unit number _____   Protocol _____

Doctor _____   Skin type _____ MED/MPD_____

Date	Treatment Number	Location			Phototherapy Record				Medications			Treatment Reactions*		Tx by	MD visit
		Body	Hand	Foot	UVB		UVA		Anthralin%	Oral	Topical	R	T		
					Time	mJ/cm^2	Time	J/cm^2							

*Treatment Reactions

Redness (R)	Tenderness/itching
0—None	0—None
1+— Fairly pink	1+— Yes/slept well
2+—Pink	2+—Yes/slept poorly
3+—Red	3+—Yes/did not sleep

SIGN AND INITIAL BELOW

OPHTHALMOLOGY EXAM RECORD

To Ophthalmologist

For Patients Being Treated With Psoralen Phototherapy

PATIENT:_____   DATE:_____

The above-mentioned patient is undergoing PUVA treatment (psoralen-ultraviolet A). An examination of the lens and retina is required of all PUVA patients. Your cooperation in recording your findings is greatly appreciated.

Please return to:

1.   Slit-lamp examination

2.   Fundoscopic examination

3.   Visual acuity

4.   Evidence of cataracts

_____ M.D.

Tel:

Address:

SELF-ADMINISTERED PSORIASIS AREA AND SEVERITY SCORING INSTRUCTIONS

The Self-Administered Psoriasis Area and Severity Index (SAPASI) provides patients with a means to objectively measure the severity of their psoriasis. The measure takes into account the area of psoriasis lesions on the body and the characteristics of these lesions—the redness, thickness, and scaliness of the lesions. Subjects shade in on a silhouette the areas that are involved. The subjects also make a mark on each of three lines to designate the redness, thickness, and scaliness of the lesions.

To score the instrument, the rater first scores the area involved for each of four areas: head, upper extremities, trunk, and lower extremities. The scoring is done on a 0–6 scale, where 0 indicates no involvement, 1 is <10%, 2 is 11%–30%, 3 is 31%–50%, 4 is 51%–70%, 5 is 71%–90%, and 6 is 91%–100%. Each of the four area scores is multiplied by a constant indicative of how large that body region is.

The head area is multiplied by 0.1, the upper extremity area by 0.2, the trunk area by 0.3, and the lower extremity area by 0.4. These normalized area scores are then summed to yield a total area score.

The color, thickness, and scale are scored by measuring in millimeters the length of the line from its beginning to the mark made by the subject. These lengths are then summed, and divided by the total length of the line in millimeters. This is multiplied by 4 to normalize each of the length scores to a 0–4 scale. Multiplying the result by the total area score yields the final SAPASI score.

To use the Scoring Sheet

1. The identifying information is completed.

2. The area scores for head, upper extremity, trunk, and lower extremity are placed in column 1, rows 1–4. The area scores are estimated using the table in the upper left-hand corner of the scoring sheet.

3. The area scores are multiplied by the corresponding values in column 2 and placed in column 3.

4. A total area score is obtained by summing the values in column 3 and placing this in row 5.

5. The color, thickness, and scaliness measurements are placed in lines 6, 7, and 8. The sum of these is placed in line 9.

6. The length of the visual analog scale is measured and placed in line 10.

7. Line 9 is divided by line 10 and placed in line 11.

8. Line 11 is multiplied by 4 and placed in line 12.

9. Line 12 is multiplied by the total area score from line 5. The result, the SAPASI score is placed in line 14.

166

The SAPASI can also be scored directly by a formula applied to the eight measured values as follows:

$$\text{SAPASI} = \left[\left(0.1 * A_H\right) + \left(0.2 * A_U\right) + \left(0.3 * A_T\right) + \left(0.4 * A_L\right)\right]$$

$$\times \left[\frac{4 * \left(\text{VAS}_E + \text{VAS}_I + \text{VAS}_S\right)}{\text{VAS}_{\text{length}}}\right]$$

where
A_H = Head area score
A_U = Upper extremity area score
A_T = Trunk area score
A_L = Lower extremities score
VAS = Visual analog scale
VAS_E = VAS erythema score (mm)
VAS_I = VAS induration score (mm)
VAS_S = VAS scale score (mm)

SELF-ADMINISTERED PSORIASIS AREA AND SEVERITY SCORING SHEET

Area scoring criteria

Score	Involvement (%)
0	None
	<10
2	11–30
3	31–50
4	51–70
5	71–90
6	91–100

IDENTIFYING INFORMATION
ID:
Name:
Date:

	Column	1	2	3
Row		Score (0–6)	Multiplier	Area Multiplier
1	Head area		0.1	
2	Upper extremity area		0.2	
3	Trunk area		0.3	
4	Lower extremity area		0.4	
5	Total area score (sum column 3, row 1–4)			

6	Color score (in millimeters)	
7	Thickness score (in millimeters)	
8	Scaliness score (in millimeters)	
9	Sum of lines 6, 7, and 8	
10	Length of visual analog scale (in millimeters)	
11	Line 9 divided by line 10	
12	4 times line 11	
13	Total area score (line 5)	
14	SAPASI score (line 11 times line 12)	

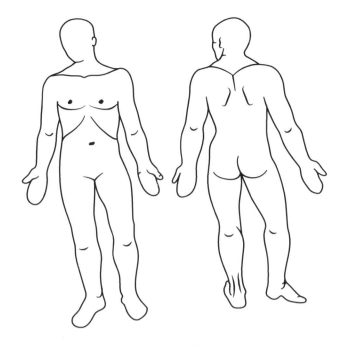

FIGURE 10.1   How bad is your psoriasis **TODAY?**

We need to know where you have psoriasis and how red, thick, and scaly it is to tell how bad your psoriasis is.

1.   As best you can, please shade in on Figure 10.1 exactly where you have psoriasis.

2.   Answer each question by placing a mark anywhere on the line to show how red, thick, and scaly an average spot of your psoriasis is (see example).

Example: How do you feel today?

_____

Good   OK   Bad   Very bad   Terrible   EXAMPLE: OK

A.   What color is an average spot of your psoriasis?

_____

No redness   Slight pink   Pink   Red   Dark red

B.   How thick is an average spot of your psoriasis?

_____

No thickness   Feels firm   Raised   Thick   Very thick

C.   How scaly is an average spot of your psoriasis?

_____

No scale   Slight scale   Scaly   Flaky   Very flaky

DOCTOR-ADMINISTERED PSORIASIS AREA AND SEVERITY SCORING INSTRUCTIONS

DATE / /	AREA	ERYTHEMA	INDURATION	SCALING
Head (H)				
Upper ext (U)				
Trunk (T)				
Lower ext (L)				

*Global overall assessment   0   1   2   3   4

DATE / /	AREA	ERYTHEMA	INDURATION	SCALING
Head (H)				
Upper ext (U)				
Trunk (T)				
Lower ext (L)				

*Global overall assessment   0   1   2   3   4

Area Scoring Score % Involvement		Erythema, Induration, and Scaling	Global Overall Assessment*
1	<10%	0 = NONE	0 = CLEAR
2	11%–30%	1 = SLIGHT	1 = MILD
3	31%–50%	2 = MODERATE	2 = MODERATE
4	51%–70%	3 = SEVERE	3 = SEVERE
5	71%–90%	4 = EXTRAORDINARILY SEVERE	4 = EXTRAORDINARILY SEVERE
6	91%–100%		

$$\text{PASI} = 0.1(E_H + I_H + S_H)A_H + 0.2(E_U + I_U + S_U)A_U + 0.3(E_T + I_T + S_T)A_T + 0.4(E_L + I_L + S_L)A_L$$

where

E = erythema

I = induration

S = scaling

A = area

FLOW SHEETS PUVA

PATIENT _____   UNIT NUMBER _____

DIAGNOSIS _____   WEIGHT:_____   PSORALEN DOSAGE _____

OPHTHALMOLOGY EXAM DATES _____   _____   _____   _____

Date													
Treatment number													
Laboratory													
Alk. phos.													
SGOT													
LDH													
Bilirubin													

COMMENTS:

_____

_____

_____

_____

_____

_____

METHOTREXATE

PATIENT _____   UNIT NUMBER _____

DIAGNOSIS   INITIAL MTX DOSAGE _____

INITIATION OF TREATMENT _____   TREATMENT ENDED _____

LABORATORY

Date														
Total bilirubin														
Alk. phos.														
SGOT														
LDH														
Protein														
WBC														
Hgb														
Hct														
Platelet														
Creatinine clearance, optional														
Baseline vital hepatitis profile														
Current MTX dosage														
Total dose to date														

LIVER BIOPSY

DATES: _____ _____ _____ _____

PATHOLOGY: _____ _____ _____ _____

RETINOID

PATIENT _____ UNIT NUMBER _____

DIAGNOSIS _____ WEIGHT _____ DOSAGE _____

INITIATION OF TREATMENT _____ TREATMENT ENDED _____

RETINOID ONLY _____ RePUVA _____

RETINOID + UVB or NBUVB _____ RETINOID+ METHOTREXATE _____

Date													
Week#													
Laboratory													
Triglyceride													
Cholesterol													
HDL													
Bilirubin													
Alk. phos.													
SGOT													
LDH													
Current dosage													
Total dose to date													

Pregnancy test (when applicable): Pas _____ Neg _____

Ophthalmology examination dates: _____ _____ _____ _____

Skeletal survey (optional): Done _____ Not done _____

Dates: _____ _____ _____ _____

CYCLOSPORINE

PATIENT NAME _____   INITIATION OF TREATMENT _____

MEDICAL RECORD# _____   TREATMENT ENDED_____

DATE											
Cyclosporine dose											
Blood pressure											
Creatinine											
BUN											
Mg											
Uric acid											
Cholesterol											
Triglyceride											
Total bilirubin											
SGOT											
Alk. phos.											
LDH											
Protein											
Na, Cl, K											
Urinalysis											
Creatinine clearance, optional											
WBC											
Hgb											
Hct											
Platelet											

A common method for determining initial and subsequent UV exposure dose is to estimate a "skin type." This method is less accurate than taking minimum erythema dose (MED) measurements.

To determine a skin type, ask the patient about his response to 30 minutes of noontime sunlight at the beginning of the summer. Skin types V and VI are based on the examination of the skin.

Skin Type	History	Examination
I	Always burns, never tans	
II	Always burns, sometimes tans	
III	Sometimes burns, always tans	
IV	Never burns, always tans	
V		Brown[a]
VI		Black

Source: Adapted from Morison, W.L., *Phototherapy and Photochemotherapy of Skin Disease*, 2nd edn., Raven Press, New York, 1991.

[a] Chinese, Mexican, American Indian.

In addition, certain medications may cause increased photosensitivity, thus affecting the initial skin type. For example, a patient normally classified as a skin type III who is also taking furosemide may actually need to be treated as a skin type II. Patient information about sensitivity to chronic sun exposure is also important. Of two patients with equal skin types, the patient who tans more slowly over time may need to be treated less aggressively.

PROCEDURE FOR DETERMINATION OF THE MINIMAL ERYTHEMA DOSE (MED) FOR UVB

1. Prior to the initiation of phototherapy treatments, the patient will be asked to attend the treatment center for 2 consecutive days.

2. The area to be tested is to be a sun-protected region on the hip or buttocks.

3. Other areas of the skin must be covered with layers of cloth over clothing or UV protective material.

4. The ports to be irradiated should be uniform in size and at least 2 cm^2.

5. Specific garments for MED determinations with eight or more ports should be used for the phototesting.

6. The location of each port should be identified by a lateral ink mark or some other type of identification for localization of the areas tested.

7. The dose for each port for routine UVB phototesting is dependent on the skin type of the person to be tested. The two dosage schedules are as follows:

Skin Types I–III (mJ/cm²)	Skin Types IV–VI (mJ/cm²)
A. 20	A. 60
B. 30	B. 70
C. 40	C. 80
D. 50	D. 90
E. 60	E. 100
F. 80	F. 120

8. The patient is to wear eye protection during the delivery of the UV doses for the MED testing.

9. The dosage delivery can best be done by beginning with all of the ports open for UV testing and closing the individual ports after a specific dose of UV light has been delivered.

10. At the completion of the phototesting, the special garments used in the testing should be removed and the areas rechecked to make sure adequate marking of the skin has been done to identify the actual ports tested.

11. The patient will be instructed not to receive any natural or artificial UV light to this region of the skin during the next 24 hours.

12. The patient is to return to the phototherapy center in 24 hours.

13. The area of the phototesting should be identified by the markings at the different dosage sites.

14. A positive reading is considered as identifiable erythema within the margins of the phototesting port.

15. If bright red erythema develops or blistering occurs at the site of any of the phototesting sites, then topical corticosteroids can be used to treat the area.

PROCEDURE FOR DETERMINATION OF THE MINIMAL ERYTHEMA DOSE (MED) FOR NARROWBAND UVB

1. Prior to the initiation of phototherapy treatments, the patient will be asked to attend the treatment center for 2 consecutive days.

2. The area to be tested is to be a sun-protected region on the hip or buttocks.

3. Other areas of the skin must be covered with layers of cloth over clothing or UV protective material.

4. The ports to be irradiated should be uniform in size and at least 2 cm².

5. Specific garments for MED determinations with six or more ports should be used for the phototesting.

6. The location of each port should be identified by a lateral ink mark or some other type of identification for localization of the areas tested.

7. The dose for each port for routine UVB phototesting is dependent on the skin type of the person to be tested. The two dosage schedules are as follows:

Skin Types I–III (mJ/cm²)	Skin Types IV–VI (mJ/cm²)
A. 400	A. 800
B. 600	B. 1000
C. 800	C. 1200
D. 1000	D. 1400
E. 1200	E. 1600
F. 1400	F. 1800

8. The patient is to wear eye protection during the delivery of the UV doses for the MED testing.

9. The dosage delivery can best be done by beginning with all of the ports open for UV testing and closing the individual ports after a specific dose of UV light has been delivered.

10. At the completion of the phototesting, the special garments used in the testing should be removed and the areas rechecked to make sure adequate marking of the skin has been done to identify the actual ports tested.

11. The patient will be instructed not to receive any natural or artificial UV light to this region of the skin during the next 24 hours.

12. The patient is to return to the phototherapy center in 24 hours.

13. The area of the phototesting should be identified by the markings at the different dosage sites.

14. A positive reading is considered as identifiable erythema within the margins of the phototesting port.

15. If bright red erythema develops or blistering occurs at the site of any of the phototesting sites, then topical corticosteroids can be used to treat the area.

DIFFERENTIAL DIAGNOSIS (TABLES A.1 THROUGH A.8)

Table A.1 Differential Diagnosis of Psoriasis: Plaque Psoriasis Vulgaris

Nummular eczema
Neurodermatitis
Tinea corporis
Lichen planus
Lupus erythematosus
Parapsoriasis
Mycosis fungoides
Bowen's squamous carcinoma
Hyperkeratotic basal cell carcinoma
Acrodermatitis enteropathica
Pityriasis rubra pilaris

Table A.2 Differential Diagnosis of Psoriasis: Flexural Psoriasis

Seborrheic eczema
Diaper dermatitis (children)
Tinea cruris
Candidiasis
Langerhan's cell histiocytosis
Perineal Bowen's carcinoma
Acrodermatitis enteropathica

Table A.3 Differential Diagnosis of Psoriasis: Guttate Psoriasis

Pityriasis rosea
Nummular eczema
Drug eruptions
Secondary syphilis
Parapsoriasis, small plaque
Cutaneous T-cell lymphoma

Table A.4 Differential Diagnosis of Psoriasis: Exfoliative Psoriasis

Eczema
  Atopic dermatitis
  Seborrheic dermatitis
  Other "endogenous" eczemas
  Contact allergic eczemas
Drug eruptions
Idiopathic
Pityriasis rubra pilaris
Pityriasis rosea
Photosensitivity skin diseases
Cutaneous lymphomas
Systemic lymphomas
Internal malignancy
Toxic epidermal necrolysis
Lichen planus
Pemphigus
Ichthyosiform erythrodermas

Table A.5 Differential Diagnosis of Psoriasis: Nail Psoriasis

Tinea unguium
Candidiasis
Trauma
Alopecia areata
Lichen planus
Drug-induced onycholysis
Twenty-nail dystrophy
Darier's disease

Table A.6 Differential Diagnosis of Psoriasis: Scalp Psoriasis

Seborrheic eczema
Tinea capitis
Pityriasis amiantacea
Lupus erythematosus
Carcinoma *in situ*
Drug eruptions
Pityriasis rubra pilaris

Table A.7 Differential Diagnosis of Psoriasis: Palmar-Plantar Psoriasis

Eczematous dermatitis
   Endogenous
   Contact allergic
Tinea manum and pedis
Reiter's syndrome
Secondary syphilis
Scabies
Cutaneous T-cell lymphoma
Acrodermatitis enteropathica

Table A.8 Differential Diagnosis of Psoriasis: Generalized Pustular Psoriasis (GPP)

Impetigo herpetiformis in pregnancy (probably variant of GPP)
Subcomeal pustular dermatosis
Pustular drug eruptions
Acrodermatitis enteropathica
Hypocalcemia

Source: Adapted from Lowe, N., *Practical Psoriasis Therapy*, 1st edn., Year Book Medical Publishers, Chicago, IL, 1986.

SOME AGENTS THAT MAY CAUSE PHOTOSENSITIVITY

Acne medications
  Tretinoin (Retin-A)

Anticancer drugs
  Dacarbazine (OTIC-Dome)
  Fluorouracil (Fluoroplex; and others)
  Methotrexate (Mexate; and others)
  Procarbazine (Matulane)
  Vinblastine (Velban)

Antidepressants
  Amitriptyline (Elavil; and other)
  Amoxapine (Asendin)
  Desipramine (Norpramin; Pertofrane)
  Doxepin (Adapin; Sinequan)
  Imipramine (Tofranil; and others)
  Isocarboxazid (Marpian)
  Maprotiline (Ludiornil)
  Nortriptyline (Aventyl; Pamelor)
  Protriptyline (Vivactil)
  Trimipramine (Surmontil)

Antihistamines
  Cyproheptadine (Periactin)
  Diphenhydramine (Benadryl; and others)

Antimicrobials
  Demeclocycline[a] (Declomycin; and others)
  Doxycycline (Vibramycin; and others)
  Griseofulvin (Fulvicin-U/F; and others)
  Methacycline (Rondomycin)
  Minocycline (Minocin)
  Nalidixic acid[a] (NegGram; and others)
  Oxytetracyclines (Terramycin; and others)
  Sulfacytine (Renoquid)
  Sulfadoxine-pyrimethamine (Fansidar)
  Sulfamethazine (Neotrizine; and others)
  Sulfamethizole (Thiosulfil; and others)
  Sulfamethoxazole (Gantanol; and others)
  Sulfamethoxazole-trimethoprim (Bactrim, Septra)
  Sulfasalazine (Azulfidine; and others)
  Sulfathiazole
  Sulfisoxazole (Gantrisin; and others)
  Tetracyclines (Achromycin; Minocin)

Antiparasitic drugs
  Bithionol (Bitin)[a]

Pyrvinium pamoate (Povan)
Quinine (many manufacturers)

Antipsychotic drugs
  Chlorpromazine (Thorazine; and others)
  Chlorprothixine (Taractan)
  Fluphenazine (Permitil; Profixin)
  Haloperidol (Haldol)
  Perphenazine (Trilafon)
  Piperacetazine (Quide)
  Prochlorperazine (Compazine; and others)
  Promethazine (Phenergen; and others)
  Thioridazine
  Thiothixene (Mellaril)
  Trifluoperazine (Stelazine; and others)
  Triflupromazine (Vesprin)
  Trimeprazine (Temaril)

Diuretics
  Acetazolamine (Diamox)
  Amiloride (Midamor)
  Bendroflumethiazide (Naturetin; and others)
  Benzthiazide (Exna; and others)
  Chlorothiazide (Diuril; and others)
  Cyclothiazide (Anhydron)
  Furosemide (Lasix)
  Hydrochlorothiazide (HydroDIURIL; and others)
  Hydroflumethiazide (Diucardin; and others)
  Methyclothiazide (Aquatensen; Enduron)
  Metolazone (Diulo; Zaroxolyn)
  Polythiazide (Renese)
  Quinethazone (Hydromox)
  Trichlormethiazide (Metahydrin; and others)
  Thiazides (Diuril; HydroDIURIL)

Hypoglycemics
  Acetohexamide (Dymelor)
  Chlorpropamide (Diabinese; Insulase)
  Glipizide (Glucotrol)
  Glyburide (DiaBeta; Micronase)
  Tolazamide (Tolinase)
  Tolbutamide (Orinase; and others)

Non-steroidal anti-inflammatory drugs
  Ketoprofen (Orudis)

Naproxen (Naprosyn)
Phenylbutazone (Butazolidin; and others)
Piroxicam (Feldene)
Sulindac (Clinoril)
Others
　Amiodarone (Cordarone)[a]
　Bergamot oil, oils of citron, lavendar, lime,
sandalwood, cedar (used in many
perfumes and cosmetics, also topical
exposure to citrus rind oils)[a]
Benzocaine
Captopril (Capoten)
Carbamazepine (Tegretol)

Source: Reprinted from Westwood Pharmaceuticals, Inc., Buffalo, NY, Copyright 1989. With permission.

Note: No sunscreen can guarantee protection from a photosensitive reaction when using any of these drugs.

[a] Reactions occur frequently.

EQUIPMENT MANUFACTURERS (NOT EXCLUSIVE)

Arjo, Inc.
50 North Gary Ave.
Unit A
Roselle, IL 60172
(800) 323-1245
www.arjo.com

Atlantic Ultraviolet Corporation
375 Marcus Blvd.
Hauppauge, NY 11788
(631) 273-0500
www.ultraviolet.com

Daavlin Corporation
PO Box 626
Bryan, OH 43506
(800) 322-8546
www.daavlin.com

Derma Light Systems (uvatec)
13425 Ventura Blvd, Suite 101
Sherman Oaks, CA 91423
(800) 882-8321
uvatec@yahoo.com

International Light, Inc.
17 Graf Road
Newburyport, MA 01950-4092
(978) 465-5923
www.intl-light.com
ilsales@intl-light.com

KBD, Inc.
2550 American Ct.
Crescent Springs, KT 41017
(800) 544-3757
www.sperti.com

Kelsun Distributors
13000 Bel-Red Road, # 206
Bellevue, WA 98005
(800) 223-3808
www.kelsun.com

National Biological Corporation
1532 Enterprise Pkwy.
Twinsburg, OH 44087
(800) 338-5045
www.natbiocorp.com

PhotoTherapeutix
1103 E. Amelia St.
Orlando, FL 32803
(407) 835-1444
www.uvbiotek.com

Psoralite Corporation
2806 Tuller Blvd.
Columbia, SC 29205
(800) 331-3534
psoralite@aol.com

The Richmond Light Co.
2301 Fallkirk Dr.
Richmond, VA 23236
(804) 276-0559
www.trlc.com

LETTER FOR HOME PHOTOTHERAPY TREATMENT

Re: NCBH#

Dear

It has been sometime since we saw you to follow up on your home phototherapy treatments. You should see your dermatologist every six months to evaluate your skin condition, any possible damage to your skin from the ultraviolet light treatments, and the need for continued treatment. If you have not seen your dermatologist in the last six months, you should stop using your home UV box.

Home ultraviolet treatments may have side effects such as allergic reactions, burning of the skin, a possible increased risk of skin cancer, increased aging of the skin, including wrinkles, freckles, loss of skin tone, and color changes, and other less common side effects. Therefore follow-up treatments are recommended for your protection.

Please feel free to call our office if you have any questions or need to schedule an appointment.

Sincerely,
cc: Chart

SUGGESTED READING

Frain-Bell W. *Cutaneous Photobiology*. Oxford, U.K.: Oxford University Press, 1985.

Harber LC, Bickers DR. *Photosensitivity Diseases. Principles of Diagnosis and Treatment*, 2nd edn. Toronto, Ontario, Canada: B.C. Decker, Inc., 1989.

Hawk JLM. *Photodermatology*. London, U.K.: Arnold, 1999.

Krutman J, Honigsmann H, Elmets CA, Bergstrasser PR. *Dermatological Phototherapy and Photodiagnostic Methods*. Berlin, Germany: Springer-Verlag, 2001.

Lim HW, Soter NA. *Clinical Photomedicine*. New York: Marcel Dekker, Inc., 1993.

Lowe N. *Practical Psoriasis Therapy*, 1st edn. Chicago, IL: Year Book Medical Publishers, 1986.

Morison WL. *Phototherapy and Photochemotherapy of Skin Disease*, 2nd edn. New York: Raven Press, 1991.